EVIDENCE-BASED ONCOLOGY FOR PRIMARY CARE PROVIDERS

EVIDENCE-BASED ONCOLOGY
FOR PRIMARY CARE PROVIDERS

Copyright © 2024 by Huynh Wynn Tran

Cover: Artist Dinh Khai - Book designer: Tien Minh Nguyen

United Buddhist Publisher (UBF)

First printed in California, USA, October 2024

ISBN-13: 979-8-3304-8333-4

© All rights reserved. No part of this book may be reproduced by any means without prior written permission.

HUYNH WYNN TRAN, MD, FACP, FACR

EVIDENCE-BASED ONCOLOGY
FOR PRIMARY CARE PROVIDERS

UBP UNITED BUDDHIST PUBLISHER

This book is dedicated to all the cancer patients I have encountered and learned from throughout my physician journey. Each of you has shaped my understanding of this disease and inspired my commitment to improving cancer care.

Most of all, this book is dedicated to my dear friend, Thuy Thanh Truong (Thuy Muoi), Founder of the Salt Cancer Initiative (SCI) in Vietnam. Your strength, vision, and dedication continue to inspire me and many others in the fight against cancer.

Preface

As the population ages, the burden of cancer is expected to grow, placing an increasing demand on primary care providers (PCPs) to manage various aspects of cancer care.

While oncologists lead the specialized treatment of cancer, PCPs play a crucial role in the early detection, management, and support of patients throughout their cancer journey. From screening and diagnosis to managing treatment side effects and coordinating care, the involvement of PCPs is vital for improving patient outcomes and quality of life.

This book is designed to provide primary care providers with a comprehensive understanding of the basics of cancer care. It covers essential topics such as the most common types of cancer, standard treatment modalities, management of complications, and cancer care nutrition. Additionally, the book explores alternative therapies and the evolving role of precision medicine in cancer care.

With the growing complexity of cancer treatments and the increasing need for collaborative care, this book serves as a guide to help PCPs better support their patients with cancer, whether by initiating appropriate referrals, managing treatment side effects, or providing nutritional, emotional, and palliative care.

By understanding cancer from a multidisciplinary perspective, PCPs can ensure that their patients receive holistic, patient-centered care throughout their cancer journey

Huynh Wynn Tran, MD, FACP, FACR
Associated Professor of Medicine and Pharmacy
CEO/Founder of Wynn Medical Center Clinics
Los Angeles, California, USA

CONTENTS

Preface 7
Part 1: Cancer and Primary Care 19
  Chapter 1: Oncology Overview for Primary Care Providers 21
    1.1. Understanding Cancer 21
      1.1.1. Genetic Mutations in Cancer 21
      1.1.2. The Tumor Microenvironment (TME) 22
      1.1.3. Metastasis 23
      1.1.4. Classification of Cancers 23
    1.2. The Role of the Primary Care Provider (PCP) in Oncology 24
      1.2.1. Cancer Prevention 24
      1.2.2. Cancer Screening 25
      1.2.3. Initial Cancer Diagnosis 26
      1.2.4. Referral to Specialists 26
      1.2.5. Follow-Up Care and Survivorship 27
    1.3. Navigating the Oncology Healthcare System 27
      1.3.1. The Multidisciplinary Care Model 28
      1.3.2. Coordination Between PCPs, Oncologists, Surgeons, and Other Specialists 28
      1.3.3. Navigating Health Systems and Resources 29
  Chapter 2: Cancer Screening and Prevention in Primary Care 31
    2.1. Evidence-Based Screening Guidelines (NCCN) 31
      2.1.1. Breast Cancer 31
      2.1.2. Colorectal Cancer 32
      2.1.3. Prostate Cancer 32
      2.1.4. Lung Cancer 33
      2.1.5. Cervical Cancer 33
      2.1.6. Skin Cancer 34
    2.2. Primary Prevention Strategies 34
      2.2.1. Lifestyle Modifications 34
      2.2.2. Vaccinations (HPV and Hepatitis B) 36
    2.3 .Risk Reduction in High-Risk Populations 36
      2.3.1. Genetic Counseling 37
      2.3.2. Chemoprevention 37
  Chapter 3: Diagnostic Approach to Suspected Cancer in Primary Care 41
    3.1. Recognizing the Red Flags Symptoms of Cancer 41
      3.1.1. Common Presenting Symptoms of Cancer 41
      3.1.2. Warning Signs for Specific Cancers 42
    3.2. Initial Cancer Diagnostic Workup 43
      3.2.1. Laboratory Tests 43
      3.2.2. Diagnostic Imaging 44
      3.2.3. Referral for Biopsy and Histopathological Examination 46

3.3. Referral to Oncology	46
3.3.1. Criteria for Timely Referrals and Pre-Referral Workup	46
3.3.2. Communicating Findings with Patients and Ensuring Follow-Up	47
Chapter 4: Cancer Staging Systems and Their Clinical Implications	51
4.1. Cancer Staging Overview (NCCN)	51
4.1.1. TNM (Tumor, Node, Metastasis) System	51
4.1.2. Prognostic Implications of TNM	52
4.1.3. Example Staging Breakdown for Common Cancers	52
4.2. Role of PCPs in Staging and Prognosis	53
4.2.1. Discussing Prognosis with Patients	54
4.2.2. Helping Patients Understand Treatment Options Based on Stage	55
Chapter 5: Evidence-Based Treatment Modalities for Cancer	57
5.1. Surgery	57
5.1.1. Curative Surgery	57
5.1.2. Palliative Surgery	58
5.1.3. Comparison of Curative and Palliative Approaches	59
5.2. Radiation Therapy	59
5.2.1. Indications for Radiation Therapy	59
5.2.2. Common Side Effects of Radiation Therapy	60
5.2.3. Advances in Radiation Therapy Technology	61
5.3. Chemotherapy	62
5.3.1. Common Chemotherapy Drugs and Regimens	62
5.3.2. Monitoring for Chemotherapy Toxicity	63
5.3. Immunotherapy	65
5.3.1. Checkpoint Inhibitors	65
5.3.2. CAR-T Cell Therapy	66
5.4. Targeted Therapy	67
5.4.1. Mechanism of Action: Targeting Cancer-Specific Molecules	67
5.4. 2. Types of Targeted Therapies	68
5.4.3. Specific Targeted Treatments	69
5.4.4. Challenges and Future Directions in Targeted Therapy	69
5.5. Hormonal Therapy	70
5.5.1. Hormonal Therapy for Breast Cancer	70
5.5.2. Hormonal Therapy for Prostate Cancer	71
5.6. Precision Medicine in Cancer Care	72
5.6.1. An Overview of Precision Medicine	72
5.6.2. Molecular Profiling and Personalized Treatment Plans	73
5.6.3. Advantages of Precision Medicine in Cancer Care	74
5.6.4. Challenges in Precision Medicine	75
5.7. Latest Advances in Cancer Treatment	75
5.7.1. Antibody-Drug Conjugates (ADCs)	75

    5.7.2. mRNA Vaccines and Their Potential Role in Oncology — 76

Part II: NCCN Cancer Treatment Guidelines — **79**
- Chapter 6: NCCN Treatment Guidelines for Common Cancers — 81
  - 6.1. Key Features of NCCN Guidelines: — 81
  - 6.2. Breast Cancer — 82
    - 6.2.1. Staging and Risk Stratification in Breast Cancer — 82
    - 6.2.2. Treatment Options for Breast Cancer — 82
    - 6.2.3. Latest Advances in Breast Cancer Treatment — 84
  - 6.3. Lung Cancer — 85
    - 6.3.1. Non-Small Cell Lung Cancer (NSCLC) — 85
    - 6.3.2. Small Cell Lung Cancer (SCLC) — 86
    - 6.3.3. Latest Advances in Lung Cancer Treatment — 87
  - 6.4. Colorectal Cancer — 87
    - 6.4.1. Screening for Colorectal Cancer — 88
    - 6.4.2. Treatment Options for Colorectal Cancer — 89
    - 6.4.3. Latest Updates in Colorectal Cancer Treatment — 90
  - 6.5. Prostate Cancer — 90
    - 6.5.1. Localized Prostate Cancer — 90
    - 6.5.2. Metastatic Prostate Cancer — 92
    - 6.5.3. Latest Updates in Prostate Cancer Treatment — 93
  - 6.6. Cervical Cancer — 93
    - 6.6.1. Screening for Cervical Cancer — 93
    - 6.6.2. Treatment Options for Cervical Cancer — 94
    - 6.6.3. Latest Advances in Cervical Cancer Treatment — 95
  - 6.7. Ovarian Cancer — 96
    - 6.7.1. Screening for Ovarian Cancer — 96
    - 6.7.2. Treatment of Ovarian Cancer: NCCN Guidelines — 97
    - 6.7.3. Latest Advances in Ovarian Cancer Treatment — 98
  - 6.8. Pancreatic Cancer — 99
    - 6.8.1. Screening for Pancreatic Cancer — 99
    - 6.8.2. Treatment of Pancreatic Cancer: NCCN Guidelines — 100
    - 6.8.3. Treatment of Unresectable and Metastatic Disease — 101
    - 6.8.4. Latest Advances in Pancreatic Cancer Treatment — 102
  - 6.9. Bladder Cancer — 102
    - 6.9.1. Screening for Bladder Cancer — 102
    - 6.9.2. Treatment of Bladder Cancer: NCCN Guidelines — 103
    - 6.9.3. Latest Advances in Bladder Cancer Treatment — 104
  - 6.10. Kidney Cancer — 105
    - 6.10.1. Screening for Kidney Cancer — 105
    - 6.10.2. Treatment of Kidney Cancer: NCCN Guidelines — 106
    - 6.10.3. Latest Advances in Kidney Cancer Treatment — 107

- 6.11. Liver Cancer (Hepatocellular Carcinoma) — 108
  - 6.11.1. Screening for Liver Cancer — 108
  - 6.11.2. Risk Factors for Liver Cancer — 109
  - 6.11.3. Treatment of Liver Cancer: NCCN Guidelines — 110
  - 6.11.4. Latest Updates in Liver Cancer Treatment — 112
- 6.12. Esophageal Cancer — 112
  - 6.12.1. Screening for Esophageal Cancer — 112
  - 6.12.2. Risk Factors for Esophageal Cancer — 113
  - 6.12.3. Treatment of Esophageal Cancer: NCCN Guidelines — 114
  - 6.12.4. Latest Advances in Esophageal Cancer Treatment — 115
- 6.13. Gastric Cancer — 116
  - 6.13.1. Screening for Gastric Cancer — 116
  - 6.13.2. Risk Factors for Gastric Cancer — 117
  - 6.13.3. Treatment of Gastric Cancer: NCCN Guidelines — 118
  - 6.13.4. Latest Advances in Gastric Cancer Treatment — 119
- 6.14. Melanoma — 120
  - 6.14.1. Screening for Melanoma — 120
  - 6.14.2. Risk Factors for Melanoma — 121
  - 6.14.3. Treatment of Melanoma: NCCN Guidelines — 122
  - 6.14.4. Latest Advances in Melanoma Treatment — 123
- 6.15. Non-Hodgkin Lymphoma — 124
  - 6.15.1. Screening for Non-Hodgkin Lymphoma — 124
  - 6.15.2. Risk Factors for Non-Hodgkin Lymphoma — 125
  - 6.15.3. Treatment of Non-Hodgkin Lymphoma: NCCN Guidelines — 126
  - 6.15.4. Latest Advances in NHL Treatment — 127
- 6.16. Hodgkin Lymphoma — 128
  - 6.16.1. Screening for Hodgkin Lymphoma — 128
  - 6.16.2. Risk Factors for Hodgkin Lymphoma — 129
  - 6.16.3. Treatment of Hodgkin Lymphoma: NCCN Guidelines — 130
  - 6.16.4. Latest Advances in Hodgkin Lymphoma Treatment — 132
- 6.17. Leukemia (Chronic and Acute) — 132
  - 6.17.1. Screening for Leukemia — 133
  - 6.17.2. Risk Factors for Leukemia — 133
  - 6.17.3. Treatment of Leukemia: NCCN Guidelines — 134
  - 6.17.4. Latest Advances in Leukemia Treatment — 136
- 6.18. Multiple Myeloma — 137
  - 6.18.1. Screening for Multiple Myeloma — 137
  - 6.18.2. Risk Factors for Multiple Myeloma — 138
  - 6.18.3. Treatment of Multiple Myeloma: NCCN Guidelines — 138
  - 6.18.4. Latest Advances in Multiple Myeloma Treatment — 140
- 6.19. Endometrial Cancer — 140

- 6.19.1. Screening for Endometrial Cancer — 140
- 6.19.2. Risk Factors for Endometrial Cancer — 141
- 6.19.3. Treatment of Endometrial Cancer: NCCN Guidelines — 142
- 6.19.4. Latest Advances in Endometrial Cancer Treatment — 144
- 6.20. Head and Neck Cancers — 144
  - 6.20.1. Screening for Head and Neck Cancer — 144
  - 6.20.2. Risk Factors for Head and Neck Cancer — 145
  - 6.20.3. Treatment of Head and Neck Cancer: NCCN Guidelines — 146
  - 6.20.4. Latest Advances in Head and Neck Cancer Treatment — 148
- 6.21. Thyroid Cancer — 148
  - 6.21.1. Screening for Thyroid Cancer — 149
  - 6.21.2. Risk Factors for Thyroid Cancer — 149
  - 6.21.3. Treatment of Thyroid Cancer: NCCN Guidelines — 150
  - 6.21.4. Latest Advances in Thyroid Cancer Treatment — 152

Chapter 7: Managing Cancer Treatment Side Effects — 157
- 7.1. Chemotherapy-Induced Side Effects — 157
  - 7.1.1. Common Chemotherapy-Induced Side Effects — 157
- 7.2. Immunotherapy-Related Side Effects (Immune-Related Adverse Events, IRAEs) — 158
- 7.3. Long-Term Side Effects of Cancer Treatment — 159

Chapter 8: Oncologic Emergencies — 161
- 8.1. Recognition and Initial Management of Oncologic Emergencies — 161
  - 8.1.1. Hypercalcemia of Malignancy — 161
  - 8.1.2. Tumor Lysis Syndrome (TLS) — 162
  - 8.1.3. Spinal Cord Compression — 162
  - 8.1.4. Febrile Neutropenia — 163
- 8.2. The PCP Can Play an Important Role — 164
  - 8.2.1. Hypercalcemia of Malignancy — 164
  - 8.2.2. Tumor Lysis Syndrome (TLS) — 164
  - 8.2.3. Spinal Cord Compression — 165
  - 8.2.4. Febrile Neutropenia — 165
- 8.3. Coordinating Care With Other Specialists — 165

Chapter 9: Palliative and End-of-Life Care in Oncology — 169
- 9.1. Integrating Palliative Care Early — 169
  - 9.1.1. Rationale for Early Integration of Palliative Care — 169
  - 9.1.2. Symptom Management in Palliative Care — 169
- 9.2. Quality of Life Discussions — 170
- 9.3. End-of-Life Conversations — 171

Chapter 10: Becoming A Cancer Survivor — 173
- 10.1. Post-Cancer Care Plans — 173
  - 10.1.1. Monitoring for Recurrence — 173
  - 10.1.2. Managing Long-Term Side Effects — 173

    10.1.3. Mental Health Support   174
  10.2 Coordination with Oncology for Long-Term Surveillance   174
    10.2.1. Importance of Coordinated Care   174
    10.2.2. Roles of the PCP and Oncologist   175
    10.2.3. Transitioning to Primary Care for Survivorship   175

Part III: Beyond Cancer Care   **177**

  Chapter 11: Chronic Pain Management in Cancer Care   179
    14.1. Pathophysiology of Cancer Pain   179
    14.2. Assessment of Chronic Cancer Pain   179
    14.3. Pharmacologic Management of Chronic Cancer Pain   180
      14.3.1. Non-Opioid Analgesics (Step 1 of the WHO Ladder)   180
      14.3.2. Opioid Analgesics (Step 2 and 3 of the WHO Ladder)   181
      14.3.3. Adjuvant Analgesics (Used Across All Steps of the WHO Ladder)   182
    14.4. Nonpharmacologic Approaches to Cancer Pain   183
      14.4.1. Physical Therapy and Rehabilitation   183
      14.4.2. Cognitive Behavioral Therapy (CBT)   184
      14.4.3. Integrative Approaches: Acupuncture, Massage Therapy, and Mindfulness   184
    14.5. Managing Opioid Side Effects and Risks   185
      14.5.1. Managing Common Opioid Side Effects   185
      14.5.2. Preventing Opioid Misuse in Cancer Patients   186
  Chapter 12: The Psychological Impact of Cancer on Patients and Family Members   189
    12.1.Psychological Impact on Cancer Patients   189
      12.1.1. Emotional Responses to a Cancer Diagnosis   189
      12.1.2. Cancer-Related Cognitive Impairment ("Chemo Brain")   190
    12.2. Psychological Impact on Family Members   190
      12.2.1. Emotional Distress and Caregiver Burden   190
      12.2.2. Impact on Family Dynamics and Relationships   191
      12.2.3. Psychological Support for Patients and Families   191
  Chapter 13: The Impact of Culture on Cancer Care   195
    13.1. Cultural Perceptions of Cancer   195
      13.1.1 Cancer as a Stigma   195
      13.1.2 Cultural Beliefs about the Causes of Cancer   195
    13.2. Impact of Culture on Cancer Screening and Prevention   196
      12.2.1 Barriers to Cancer Screening   196
      13.2.2 Cultural Influences on Health-Seeking Behaviors   196
    13.3. Cultural Differences in Cancer Treatment Decision-Making   197
      13.3.1 Individualism vs. Collectivism in Decision-Making   197
      13.3.2 Truth-Telling and Disclosure of Prognosis   197
    13.4. Culture and End-of-Life Care in Cancer   198
      13.4.1 Preferences for Life-Sustaining Treatments   198

13.4.2 Cultural and Religious Beliefs About Death	198
Chapter 14: Supplements and Vitamins in Cancer: What is the Evidence?	201
14.1. Overview of Supplement Use in Cancer Patients	201
1.1 Prevalence of Supplement Use	201
1.2 Reasons for Supplement Use	201
14.2. Evidence-Based Review of Common Supplements and Vitamins in Cancer Care	201
14.2.1 Antioxidants (Vitamin C, Vitamin E, Beta-Carotene)	201
14.2.2 Vitamin D	202
14.2.3 Omega-3 Fatty Acids	203
14.2.4 Curcumin (Turmeric)	203
14.3. Risks and Concerns with Supplement Use in Cancer	204
14.3.1 Interference with Conventional Treatments	204
14.3.2 Lack of Regulation and Quality Control	204
14.4. Guidelines for Healthcare Providers and Patients	204
14.4.1. Open Communication	204
14.4.2. Assess for Drug-Supplement Interactions	205
14.4.3. Evidence-Based Recommendations for Supplement Use	206
14.4.4. Focus on Nutrition	206
Chapter 15: Exercise and Cancer Care	209
15.1. Exercise and Cancer Prevention	209
15.1.1 Evidence for Cancer Prevention	209
15.1.2 Mechanisms of Action	209
15.2. Exercise During Cancer Treatment	210
15.2.1 Benefits of Exercise During Treatment	210
15.2.2 Safety Considerations	211
15.3. Exercise and Cancer Survivorship	211
15.3.1 Benefits of Exercise for Cancer Survivors	211
15.3.2 Recommendations for Cancer Survivors	212
15.4. Integrating Exercise into Cancer Care	212
15.4.1 The Role of Healthcare Providers	212
15.4.2 Barriers to Exercise in Cancer Care	212
Chapter 16: Nutrition in Cancer Care: Evidence for Primary Care Providers (PCPs)	215
16.1. The Role of Nutrition in Cancer Care	215
16.1.1. Malnutrition in Cancer Patients	215
16.1.2. Cancer Cachexia	216
16.1.3. Treatment-Related Side Effects and Nutritional Challenges	216
16.1.4. Importance of Early Nutritional Interventions	217
16.2. Nutritional Screening and Assessment	217
16.2.1. Nutritional Screening Tools: Identifying Patients at Risk	218
16.2.2. Components of a Comprehensive Nutritional Assessment	218

- 16.2.3. Role of Nutritional Assessment Throughout Cancer Treatment — 219
- 16.3 Nutritional Interventions During Cancer Treatment — 220
  - 16.3.1. Enteral and Parenteral Nutrition — 220
  - 16.3.2. Dietary Modifications During Chemotherapy and Radiation Therapy — 221
- 16.4. Evidence-Based Dietary Recommendations for Cancer Patients — 221
  - 16.4.1. A Plant-Based Diet: High in Fruits, Vegetables, and Whole Grains — 221
  - 16.4.2. Lean Proteins for Muscle Preservation — 222
  - 16.4.3. Healthy Fats: Omega-3 Fatty Acids and Avoidance of Trans Fats — 223
  - 16.4.4. Hydration and Managing Treatment Side Effects — 223
  - 16.4.5. Avoiding Sugar and Processed Foods — 224
- 16.5. Supporting Long-Term Survivors — 225

Appendix A: Nutritional Screening Tools — 227
1. Malnutrition Universal Screening Tool (MUST) — 227
2. Patient-Generated Subjective Global Assessment (PG-SGA) — 227
3. Simplified Nutritional Assessment Questionnaire (SNAQ) — 228

Appendix B: Dietary Recommendations by Cancer Type — 231
1. Colorectal Cancer — 231
2. Breast Cancer — 231
3. Lung Cancer — 232
4. Prostate Cancer — 233
5. Ovarian Cancer — 233
6. Pancreatic Cancer — 234

Appendix C: Guidelines for Managing Cancer Treatment Side Effects — 235
1. Nausea and Vomiting — 235
2. Diarrhea — 235
3. Mucositis (Mouth Sores) — 236
4. Taste Changes (Dysgeusia) — 237
5. Constipation — 237
6. Loss of Appetite (Anorexia) — 238

Appendix D: Pharmacological Agents for Managing Cancer-Related Symptoms — 239
1. Antiemetics: Managing Nausea and Vomiting — 239
2. Appetite Stimulants — 240
3. Pain Medications — 240
4. Laxatives and Stool Softeners: Managing Opioid-Induced Constipation (OIC) — 241
5. Corticosteroids — 242

Appendix E: Physical Activity Recommendations for Cancer Patients — 243
1. General Physical Activity Guidelines for Cancer Patients — 243
2. Special Considerations for Cancer-Related Fatigue — 243
3. Exercise Recommendations for Cancer Cachexia and Muscle Loss — 244
4. Considerations for Patients with Bone Metastases — 245
5. Exercise for Patients Undergoing Chemotherapy or Radiation Therapy — 245

    6. Flexibility and Balance Exercises — 246
Appendix F: Cancer Screening Guidelines — 247
    1. Breast Cancer — 247
    2. Colorectal Cancer — 247
    3. Lung Cancer — 248
    4. Prostate Cancer — 248
    5. Cervical Cancer — 249
    6. Ovarian Cancer — 249
    7. Endometrial Cancer — 250
    8. Melanoma — 250
    9. Liver Cancer (Hepatocellular Carcinoma) — 250

Part 1: Cancer and Primary Care

Chapter 1: Oncology Overview for Primary Care Providers

1.1. Understanding Cancer

Cancer is a complex disease characterized by the uncontrolled growth of abnormal cells, typically resulting from genetic mutations that disrupt normal cellular processes. The hallmark features of cancer include:

- **Sustained proliferative signaling**: Cancer cells continuously receive signals to divide.
- **Evasion of growth suppressors**: These cells bypass normal mechanisms that limit cell proliferation.
- **Resistance to cell death**: Cancer cells evade programmed cell death (apoptosis).
- **Replicative immortality**: These cells can divide indefinitely, unlike normal cells.
- **Induction of angiogenesis**: Tumors stimulate the growth of new blood vessels to supply nutrients.
- **Activation of invasion and metastasis**: Cancer cells spread to other tissues and organs.

These hallmarks are fundamental to understanding cancer's biology and its aggressive nature. Over the past decades, advances in molecular biology and cancer genetics have deepened our understanding of these processes, leading to new therapeutic strategies.

1.1.1. Genetic Mutations in Cancer

Genetic mutations are the primary drivers of cancer, leading to the disruption of normal cellular functions. These mutations can be categorized into two main types:

- **Germline mutations**: These are inherited mutations passed down from one generation to the next. They increase the risk of developing certain cancers, such as breast cancer (mutations in **BRCA1** and **BRCA2**) and colorectal cancer (mutations in **APC**).
- **Somatic mutations**: These are acquired mutations that occur during an individual's life due to environmental exposures (e.g., smoking, radiation) or random errors in DNA replication. Somatic mutations are the most common cause of cancer and affect genes involved in critical cellular functions.

Oncogenes and Tumor Suppressor Genes

- **Oncogenes**: Oncogenes are mutated or overexpressed genes that promote cell growth and proliferation. In their normal form, these genes are called **proto-oncogenes**. When mutated, they drive cancer progression by constantly signaling cells to grow. Examples of oncogenes include **KRAS**, **BRAF**, and **MYC**. These genes play critical roles in signaling pathways that regulate cell division and survival. For instance, mutations in **KRAS** are common in colon, lung, and pancreatic cancers, while mutations in **BRAF** are frequently found in melanoma.

- **Tumor suppressor genes**: These genes function to prevent uncontrolled cell division by regulating the cell cycle and promoting apoptosis (programmed cell death). When tumor suppressor genes are mutated, cancer cells can proliferate without regulation. Key examples include **TP53** and **RB1**. **TP53**, often referred to as the "guardian of the genome," is the most frequently mutated gene in human cancers, with alterations found in more than 50% of all tumors. **RB1** regulates the cell cycle and, when mutated, contributes to the development of retinoblastoma and other cancers.

Driver vs. Passenger Mutations

- **Driver mutations**: These mutations are directly responsible for initiating and promoting cancer development. They typically affect critical genes like oncogenes and tumor suppressor genes, leading to abnormal growth signaling, cell survival, or genomic instability.
- **Passenger mutations**: These mutations occur as byproducts of cancer development but do not contribute to the initiation or progression of the disease. They accumulate in cancer cells due to the overall genomic instability of tumors but do not influence cancer behavior.

1.1.2. The Tumor Microenvironment (TME)

The **tumor microenvironment (TME)** refers to the complex network of non-cancerous cells and extracellular components that surround and interact with cancer cells. The TME plays a critical role in tumor progression, metastasis, and response to treatment. It consists of:

- **Cancer-associated fibroblasts (CAFs)**: These cells secrete growth factors, cytokines, and extracellular matrix components that promote tumor growth and metastasis.
- **Immune cells**: Tumor-infiltrating immune cells, such as **macrophages** and **T-cells**, can either attack or support the tumor. **Tumor-associated macrophages (TAMs)**, for example, can promote tumor growth by secreting pro-inflammatory and pro-angiogenic factors.
- **Endothelial cells**: These cells line blood vessels and contribute to **angiogenesis**, the formation of new blood vessels, which supplies the tumor with oxygen and nutrients.
- **Extracellular matrix (ECM)**: The ECM provides structural support to tumors and influences cancer cell behavior by modulating cell adhesion, migration, and signaling.

The TME plays a critical role in enabling cancer cells to evade the immune system, resist therapy, and promote metastasis. Targeting the TME has become a major focus of cancer therapy development, particularly in **immuno-oncology**. For example, immune checkpoint inhibitors such as **pembrolizumab** (an anti-PD-1 antibody) work by modulating the immune response within the TME to enhance the ability of the immune system to recognize and attack cancer cells (**Topalian et al., 2012**).

1.1.3. Metastasis

Metastasis, the process by which cancer cells spread from the primary tumor site to distant organs, is responsible for the majority of cancer-related deaths. It involves several distinct steps:

- **Local invasion**: Cancer cells invade surrounding tissues.
- **Intravasation**: Cancer cells enter blood vessels or lymphatic vessels.
- **Circulation**: Cancer cells travel through the bloodstream or lymphatic system.
- **Extravasation**: Cancer cells exit the blood vessels and invade distant tissues.
- **Colonization**: Cancer cells grow and form secondary tumors at distant sites.

Key molecular processes involved in metastasis include:

- **Epithelial-Mesenchymal Transition (EMT)**: During EMT, cancer cells lose their epithelial characteristics (e.g., cell-cell adhesion) and gain mesenchymal traits (e.g., increased mobility), enabling them to invade nearby tissues and spread. EMT is regulated by transcription factors such as **Snail** and **Twist** (**Kalluri and Weinberg, 2009**).
- **Matrix Metalloproteinases (MMPs)**: MMPs are enzymes that degrade the extracellular matrix, facilitating cancer cell invasion and migration. Overexpression of MMPs has been implicated in the metastatic spread of many cancers (**Egeblad and Werb, 2002**).
- **Chemokine signaling**: Chemokines and their receptors (e.g., **CXCR4**) guide cancer cells to specific tissues where they can form metastases. For example, **CXCR4** is overexpressed in breast cancer cells and plays a key role in metastasis to the lungs and bone (**Müller et al., 2001**).

Research into metastasis has focused on finding ways to block these processes, thereby preventing the spread of cancer. Therapies that target MMPs or chemokine signaling pathways are under investigation for their potential to inhibit metastatic progression.

1.1.4. Classification of Cancers

Cancers are classified based on the type of tissue from which they originate and the characteristics of the cancer cells.

Solid Tumors

Solid tumors originate from epithelial, connective, or nervous tissues and are categorized by the organ of origin (e.g., breast, lung, prostate) and histologic subtype. Common subtypes include:

- **Adenocarcinoma**: Arising from glandular tissue, common in the breast, prostate, and lung.
- **Squamous cell carcinoma**: Originating from squamous epithelium, often found in the skin, lungs, and head and neck region.

Solid tumors can remain localized or spread to regional lymph nodes and distant organs (metastasis). Treatments often involve surgery, chemotherapy, radiation, and targeted therapies depending on the tumor stage and molecular profile.

Hematologic Cancers

Hematologic cancers involve malignancies of the blood, bone marrow, or lymphatic system. These cancers often disrupt normal blood cell production and immune function, leading to conditions such as anemia, immunosuppression, and increased susceptibility to infections. Hematologic malignancies include:

- **Leukemia**: Cancers of the bone marrow and blood that affect white blood cell production (e.g., **acute myeloid leukemia**, **chronic lymphocytic leukemia**).
- **Lymphoma**: Cancers that originate in the lymphatic system, including **Hodgkin lymphoma** and **non-Hodgkin lymphoma**.
- **Multiple myeloma**: A cancer of plasma cells in the bone marrow that affects immune function and bone integrity.

The classification of hematologic cancers is often based on the type of blood cell affected and the genetic mutations involved.

1.2. The Role of the Primary Care Provider (PCP) in Oncology

As the first point of contact for most patients, PCPs help detect cancer early, manage chronic conditions in cancer survivors, and ensure coordinated care across multiple healthcare providers.

1.2.1. Cancer Prevention

PCPs play a pivotal role in cancer prevention by promoting lifestyle changes and preventive measures that reduce the risk of cancer. Prevention is one of the most impactful roles a PCP can play in oncology, as many cancers are influenced by modifiable risk factors.

Lifestyle Counseling

PCPs provide guidance on lifestyle modifications that are crucial for cancer prevention. These include:

- **Smoking cessation**: Smoking is one of the leading causes of lung cancer and other cancers. PCPs offer counseling, nicotine replacement therapies, and pharmacologic interventions such as **varenicline** and **bupropion** to help patients quit smoking.
- **Healthy diet**: A balanced diet rich in fruits, vegetables, and whole grains has been associated with a reduced risk of various cancers. PCPs educate patients on the importance of reducing processed meats, red meats, and refined sugars, which have been linked to an increased risk of colorectal and other cancers.

- **Regular physical activity**: Physical inactivity is a known risk factor for many cancers, including breast, colon, and endometrial cancers. PCPs encourage patients to engage in at least 150 minutes of moderate-intensity exercise per week, as recommended by the **American Cancer Society (ACS)**.

HPV Vaccination

The **Centers for Disease Control and Prevention (CDC)** recommends the human papillomavirus (HPV) vaccination to prevent HPV-related cancers, including cervical, anal, and oropharyngeal cancers. The HPV vaccine has been shown to reduce the incidence of these cancers significantly. PCPs play a critical role in educating patients and parents about the importance of the vaccine, which is recommended for both males and females starting at ages 11-12, with catch-up vaccinations for adults up to age 26.

- **Studies** have shown a dramatic decline in the incidence of cervical cancer due to widespread vaccination, especially in younger populations. **Markowitz et al. (2016)** demonstrated a 64% reduction in vaccine-type HPV infections among teenage girls in the U.S. since the introduction of the vaccine.

Genetic Counseling and Testing

For patients with a family history of cancer, PCPs are responsible for assessing risk and guiding patients to genetic counseling and testing when appropriate. Genetic testing, such as for **BRCA1** and **BRCA2** mutations, can identify individuals at higher risk for breast, ovarian, and other cancers. Genetic counseling is essential to discuss the implications of testing, management options, and preventive measures such as increased surveillance, prophylactic surgery, or chemoprevention.

1.2.2. Cancer Screening

Early detection through cancer screening can drastically improve treatment outcomes, as many cancers are curable if caught in early stages. PCPs are on the frontlines of implementing evidence-based screening guidelines and ensuring that patients undergo appropriate tests based on their age, risk factors, and family history.

Screening Guidelines

PCPs follow evidence-based guidelines provided by organizations such as the **U.S. Preventive Services Task Force (USPSTF)** and the **National Comprehensive Cancer Network (NCCN)** to screen for common cancers:

- **Breast cancer**: Mammography is recommended every 1-2 years for women aged 50-74, while women with a family history or genetic predisposition may require earlier and more frequent screening.

- **Colorectal cancer**: Screening with colonoscopy, fecal immunochemical tests (FIT), or stool DNA tests is recommended starting at age 45 for average-risk individuals, with earlier screening for those with a family history.
- **Prostate cancer**: PSA testing may be offered to men aged 55-69 based on shared decision-making, weighing the benefits and potential harms of screening.
- **Lung cancer**: Low-dose CT screening is recommended for individuals aged 50-80 with a significant smoking history (20 pack-years or more) who currently smoke or have quit within the past 15 years.

Risk Stratification and High-Risk Patients

PCPs assess individual risk factors, such as genetic predispositions, lifestyle habits, and environmental exposures, to determine personalized screening schedules. For example, patients with **Lynch syndrome**, a hereditary condition that increases the risk for colorectal and other cancers, may require more frequent colonoscopies starting at a younger age. Similarly, women with **BRCA mutations** often begin breast cancer screening with both mammography and MRI at a younger age.

1.2.3. Initial Cancer Diagnosis

PCPs are often the first to evaluate patients who present with symptoms that may be indicative of cancer. Identifying "red flag" symptoms and initiating a diagnostic workup promptly is crucial to improving outcomes.

Recognizing Cancer Symptoms

Some of the common symptoms that may raise suspicion for cancer include:

- **Unexplained weight loss**: This can be a sign of cancers such as gastrointestinal, pancreatic, or lung cancer.
- **Persistent cough or hemoptysis**: May indicate lung cancer, especially in smokers.
- **Rectal bleeding**: A potential sign of colorectal cancer.
- **Palpable masses**: A lump in the breast or neck can signal breast cancer or lymphoma.

When these symptoms are identified, PCPs initiate further investigation through diagnostic imaging (e.g., X-ray, CT scan, ultrasound) and laboratory tests, including tumor markers (e.g., PSA, CEA, CA-125). Early diagnostic workups reduce the time to treatment and improve the prognosis for many cancers.

1.2.4. Referral to Specialists

When cancer is suspected or diagnosed, timely referral to the appropriate specialists is critical. PCPs play an essential role in coordinating care between oncologists, surgeons, radiation therapists, and other specialists.

Role in Multidisciplinary Care

PCPs are responsible for ensuring that patients receive comprehensive, coordinated care by facilitating referrals and communicating with oncology teams. **Multidisciplinary tumor boards**, which include oncologists, radiologists, pathologists, and other specialists, are often involved in the planning of treatment, and PCPs ensure that patients are referred to these boards when appropriate.

Palliative Care Referrals

For patients with advanced or metastatic cancer, PCPs may also help initiate **palliative care** referrals. Palliative care focuses on improving quality of life by managing symptoms such as pain, fatigue, and emotional distress. Studies have shown that early palliative care integration improves both quality of life and, in some cases, survival for patients with advanced cancer (**Temel et al., 2010**).

1.2.5. Follow-Up Care and Survivorship

PCPs play a central role in the long-term care of cancer survivors, particularly as they transition from active treatment to survivorship. Long-term care involves monitoring for cancer recurrence, managing comorbidities, and addressing the long-term side effects of cancer therapies.

Survivorship Care Plans

Survivorship care plans, developed in collaboration with oncologists, outline the follow-up care needed for cancer survivors. These plans include:

- **Surveillance for recurrence**: Regular imaging, laboratory tests, and clinical exams are critical for detecting cancer recurrence.
- **Management of late effects**: Many cancer treatments, including chemotherapy and radiation, can cause long-term side effects such as **cardiotoxicity** (e.g., from anthracyclines), **neuropathy**, and **osteoporosis**. PCPs manage these conditions and collaborate with specialists to optimize the patient's quality of life.
- **Comorbidities**: Cancer survivors often have pre-existing or treatment-induced comorbidities, such as diabetes or cardiovascular disease. PCPs monitor and treat these conditions while coordinating care with other specialists.

Mental Health and Quality of Life

Cancer survivors may experience long-term psychological challenges, including anxiety, depression, and fear of recurrence. PCPs are responsible for assessing mental health needs and referring patients to counselors, psychiatrists, or support groups as necessary. Maintaining open lines of communication and encouraging regular follow-ups are essential components of survivorship care.

1.3. Navigating the Oncology Healthcare System

Cancer care is multifaceted, requiring the involvement of numerous specialists and coordinated efforts across different stages of diagnosis, treatment, and survivorship. For optimal outcomes, a collaborative and integrated approach is crucial. Primary care providers (PCPs) play a critical role within this complex system, acting as both patient advocates and coordinators of care.

1.3.1. The Multidisciplinary Care Model

The complexity of cancer care necessitates a **multidisciplinary care model**, where a team of healthcare professionals, each with specialized expertise, collaborate to provide comprehensive care. This team often includes oncologists, surgeons, radiologists, pathologists, genetic counselors, palliative care specialists, and other healthcare providers. The goal is to create a personalized, evidence-based treatment plan that considers the unique needs of each patient.

Key Members of the Multidisciplinary Team (MDT)

- **Medical Oncologists**: Oversee systemic cancer treatments, including chemotherapy, immunotherapy, and targeted therapy.
- **Surgical Oncologists**: Perform surgeries to remove tumors and affected tissues, often playing a critical role in curative treatment plans.
- **Radiation Oncologists**: Use radiation therapy to target and kill cancer cells, either as a primary treatment or in conjunction with surgery and systemic therapies.
- **Pathologists**: Analyze tissue biopsies and blood samples to provide precise diagnoses and identify the cancer's molecular characteristics.
- **Radiologists**: Perform diagnostic imaging (CT, MRI, PET scans) to determine tumor size, spread, and treatment effectiveness.
- **Genetic Counselors**: Evaluate patients' genetic risk for hereditary cancers and provide counseling on genetic testing, such as BRCA mutation analysis.
- **Palliative Care Providers**: Focus on symptom management, improving quality of life, and addressing emotional, social, and spiritual needs, especially in advanced cancer cases.
- **Nurse Navigators/Care Coordinators**: Assist patients in navigating the healthcare system, scheduling appointments, and connecting them with resources such as support groups and financial assistance programs.

1.3.2. Coordination Between PCPs, Oncologists, Surgeons, and Other Specialists

Effective communication and collaboration between the PCP and oncology specialists are essential to delivering seamless, coordinated cancer care. Each specialist brings expertise to a specific aspect of care, but the PCP remains the central figure responsible for ensuring that the patient's overall health and well-being are managed throughout the cancer journey.

Key Responsibilities of the PCP

- **Management of Comorbid Conditions**: Many cancer patients have chronic health conditions (e.g., diabetes, heart disease) that must be carefully managed during cancer

treatment. Chemotherapy, radiation, and other therapies can exacerbate these conditions, requiring the PCP to monitor and adjust medications and treatments accordingly.
- **Monitoring Treatment Side Effects**: PCPs also help manage the side effects of cancer treatments. For example, chemotherapy can cause peripheral neuropathy, fatigue, and anemia, while radiation therapy can lead to skin damage, lung toxicity, or gastrointestinal issues. PCPs provide supportive care to alleviate these symptoms and improve the patient's quality of life.
- **Supportive Care During and After Treatment**: Beyond the management of side effects, PCPs address the psychological and emotional well-being of cancer patients, referring them to mental health services, social workers, or palliative care as needed.

1.3.3. Navigating Health Systems and Resources

Cancer care is often expensive and resource-intensive, involving a variety of services, treatments, and support mechanisms. Navigating these systems can be overwhelming for patients, especially those facing financial challenges, language barriers, or limited access to care. PCPs play a vital role in helping patients access the care and resources they need to overcome these barriers.

- **Insurance coverage**: Understanding what treatments are covered by insurance, obtaining prior authorizations, and dealing with denied claims can be complicated. PCPs and their teams assist patients in communicating with insurance companies and accessing covered services.
- **Patient assistance programs**: For patients with financial difficulties, many pharmaceutical companies offer patient assistance programs that provide medications at reduced or no cost. Additionally, cancer-specific organizations like the **American Cancer Society (ACS)** and **Leukemia & Lymphoma Society (LLS)** offer grants and resources to cover treatment-related expenses.

Access to Clinical Trials

PCPs play an essential role in guiding patients toward clinical trials that offer access to innovative therapies not yet widely available. **Clinical trials** are critical for the development of new cancer treatments, and many patients may benefit from participating, especially those with advanced or treatment-resistant cancers. PCPs, in collaboration with oncologists, help patients find appropriate trials and understand the potential risks and benefits.

- **NCI-MATCH (Molecular Analysis for Therapy Choice)** is an example of a precision medicine trial where patients are matched with treatments based on the specific genetic mutations driving their cancer. Such trials provide hope for personalized therapies that target the unique biology of each patient's cancer (**The Cancer Genome Atlas Research Network, 2013**).

Nurse Navigators and Care Coordinators

Many cancer centers and hospitals provide **nurse navigators** or **care coordinators** to guide patients through the complexities of cancer care. These professionals help patients manage their appointments, coordinate care between specialists, and ensure that treatment progresses smoothly. Nurse navigators also provide emotional support and connect patients with additional resources, such as home health services, physical therapy, or dietary counseling.

Research has shown that nurse navigators improve patient outcomes by reducing delays in care, enhancing patient satisfaction, and increasing adherence to treatment plans. For example, a study by **Case (2011)** demonstrated that nurse navigators improved treatment adherence and reduced distress among newly diagnosed cancer patients.

References

- Hanahan D, Weinberg RA. Hallmarks of cancer: the next generation. *Cell*. 2011;144(5):646-674.
- Stratton MR, Campbell PJ, Futreal PA. The cancer genome. *Nature*. 2009;458(7239):719-724.
- Vogelstein B, Papadopoulos N, Velculescu VE, et al. Cancer genome landscapes. *Science*. 2013;339(6127):1546-1558.
- Quail DF, Joyce JA. Microenvironmental regulation of tumor progression and metastasis. *Nat Med*. 2013;19(11):1423-1437.
- Schreiber RD, Old LJ, Smyth MJ. Cancer immunoediting: integrating immunity's roles in cancer suppression and promotion. *Science*. 2011;331(6024):1565-1570.
- Steeg PS. Tumor metastasis: mechanistic insights and clinical challenges. *Nat Med*. 2006;12(8):895-904.
- Kalluri R, Weinberg RA. The basics of epithelial-mesenchymal transition. *J Clin Invest*. 2009;119(6):1420-1428.
- Siegel RL, Miller KD, Fuchs HE, Jemal A. Cancer statistics, 2022. *CA Cancer J Clin*. 2022;72(1):7-33.
- Greaves M. Evolutionary determinants of cancer. *Science*. 2018;362(6411):976-978.
- Colditz GA, Wei EK. Preventability of cancer: the relative contributions of biologic and social and physical environmental determinants of cancer mortality. *Annu Rev Public Health*. 2012;33:137-156.
- Meites E, Szilagyi PG, Chesson HW, et al. Human papillomavirus vaccination for adults: updated recommendations of the Advisory Committee on Immunization Practices. *MMWR Morb Mortal Wkly Rep*. 2019;68(32):698-702.
- Nelson HD, Pappas M, Zakher B, et al. Risk assessment, genetic counseling, and genetic testing for BRCA-related cancer in women: updated evidence report and systematic review for the US Preventive Services Task Force. *JAMA*. 2019;322(7):666-685.
- U.S. Preventive Services Task Force. Screening for colorectal cancer: US Preventive Services Task Force recommendation statement. *JAMA*. 2021;325(19):1965-1977.

Chapter 2: Cancer Screening and Prevention in Primary Care

Cancer screening and prevention are integral components of oncology care, particularly in the primary care setting. Early detection through screening can lead to improved survival outcomes, and preventive measures can reduce the risk of cancer development.

Primary care providers (PCPs) play a central role in implementing evidence-based guidelines for screening and advising patients on cancer prevention strategies.

2.1. Evidence-Based Screening Guidelines (NCCN)

Cancer screening is a critical component of cancer prevention and early detection, significantly improving outcomes by identifying cancers at earlier, more treatable stages. The National Comprehensive Cancer Network (NCCN) and other leading organizations like the **American Cancer Society (ACS)** and **U.S. Preventive Services Task Force (USPSTF)** provide guidelines based on the latest research, ensuring that screening recommendations are evidence-based and tailored to patient risk factors. Below is a detailed review of the current screening guidelines for the most common cancers, with a focus on the NCCN guidelines and supporting evidence.

2.1.1. Breast Cancer

Mammography

Mammography is the gold standard for breast cancer screening and has been shown to reduce mortality, particularly in women aged 50-74. Studies, including those by the **U.S. Preventive Services Task Force (USPSTF)** and **American Cancer Society (ACS)**, have established varying recommendations for when and how often screening should occur based on age and individual risk factors.

- **USPSTF Recommendation**: Biennial screening for women aged 50-74.
- **ACS Recommendation**: Annual screening starting at age 45, with a transition to biennial screening at age 55 for women with average risk.
- **NCCN Guidelines**: Screening should be individualized, with earlier screening advised for women at higher risk, such as those with a family history of breast cancer or those with genetic predispositions like **BRCA1/2 mutations**.

Mammography has been proven to reduce mortality from breast cancer. A large study, **Miller et al. (2014)**, showed a significant reduction in breast cancer mortality in women who underwent regular mammographic screening.

Genetic Screening for BRCA1/2 Mutations

Women with a family history of early-onset breast or ovarian cancer, or male relatives with breast cancer, are advised to undergo genetic counseling and testing for **BRCA1/2 mutations**.

Carriers of these mutations face a significantly higher lifetime risk of developing breast and ovarian cancers.

- **NCCN and USPSTF Recommendations**: Both organizations recommend genetic counseling and testing for women at high risk due to personal or family history. Identifying BRCA mutation carriers enables preventive strategies, such as enhanced screening, risk-reducing surgery, or chemoprevention.

Nelson et al. (2019) reviewed risk assessment models for BRCA-related cancers and found that interventions based on genetic testing, including prophylactic mastectomy and oophorectomy, reduce cancer incidence among mutation carriers.

2.1.2. Colorectal Cancer

Colonoscopy

Colonoscopy is considered the preferred method for colorectal cancer screening as it allows for the direct visualization and removal of precancerous polyps. Studies demonstrate that regular colonoscopy screening reduces both the incidence and mortality of colorectal cancer.

- **NCCN Recommendation**: Screening should begin at age 45 for individuals at average risk, with follow-up screenings every 10 years if no abnormalities are found.
- **USPSTF**: Recommends colorectal cancer screening starting at age 45, emphasizing that both colonoscopy and other screening methods are highly effective.

A study by **Zauber et al. (2012)** found that colonoscopy was associated with a 68% reduction in the risk of dying from colorectal cancer when performed at recommended intervals.

FIT-DNA Tests (Stool-Based Tests)

Non-invasive stool-based tests, such as the **Fecal Immunochemical Test (FIT)** and **FIT-DNA (Cologuard)**, detect occult blood or abnormal DNA in the stool and are suitable for individuals who prefer non-invasive screening.

- **NCCN and USPSTF Recommendations**: Annual FIT or FIT-DNA screening every three years for individuals who choose this non-invasive method.

Imperiale et al. (2014) found that FIT-DNA testing has a high sensitivity for detecting colorectal cancer, although colonoscopy remains the gold standard due to its diagnostic and therapeutic capabilities.

2.1.3. Prostate Cancer

Prostate-Specific Antigen (PSA) Screening

Prostate cancer screening remains controversial due to concerns about overdiagnosis and overtreatment, particularly in men with indolent, slow-growing tumors. PSA-based screening requires careful consideration of the potential benefits and harms, especially for younger men at high risk.

- **USPSTF Recommendation**: Advocates shared decision-making for men aged 55-69, emphasizing that screening should reflect patient preferences and values.
- **NCCN Guidelines**: Supports PSA screening starting at age 45 for men at high risk, such as African American men or those with a family history of prostate cancer.

Shared Decision-Making

A key aspect of prostate cancer screening is shared decision-making, in which patients are fully informed of the benefits and risks of screening, including potential complications like erectile dysfunction and urinary incontinence after treatment. The **Prostate, Lung, Colorectal, and Ovarian (PLCO) Cancer Screening Trial** found that routine PSA screening did not significantly reduce mortality from prostate cancer, underscoring the need for individualized screening decisions (**Andriole et al., 2009**).

2.1.4. Lung Cancer

Low-Dose CT (LDCT) Screening

Lung cancer is the leading cause of cancer-related deaths worldwide. Early detection through **low-dose CT (LDCT)** has been shown to reduce lung cancer mortality in high-risk populations, as evidenced by the **National Lung Screening Trial (NLST)**, which demonstrated a 20% reduction in mortality with annual LDCT screening.

- **NCCN and USPSTF Recommendations**: Both recommend annual LDCT screening for individuals aged 50-80 with a 20-30 pack-year smoking history who currently smoke or have quit within the past 15 years.

Aberle et al. (2011) reported that LDCT significantly reduced lung cancer mortality compared to chest X-rays in high-risk individuals, making it the preferred screening method for early detection in smokers.

2.1.5. Cervical Cancer

Pap Smear and HPV Co-Testing

Cervical cancer screening has been one of the most successful cancer prevention measures. The introduction of **HPV testing** alongside traditional **Pap smears** has further improved the ability to detect precancerous changes.

- **USPSTF Recommendations**: Pap smears every three years for women aged 21-29, and co-testing (Pap smear + HPV test) every five years for women aged 30-65.

- **NCCN Guidelines**: Also endorse co-testing for women aged 30 and older as the preferred screening strategy.

A landmark study by **Castle et al. (2011)** found that HPV co-testing improves the accuracy of cervical cancer screening, identifying more cases of high-grade cervical intraepithelial neoplasia than Pap smears alone.

2.1.6. Skin Cancer

Screening for High-Risk Populations (ABCDE Method for Melanoma)

There are no formal recommendations for routine skin cancer screening in the general population. However, individuals at high risk, such as those with a family history of melanoma, fair skin, or significant UV exposure, should be monitored closely.

- **ABCDE Method**: The ABCDE method (Asymmetry, Border irregularity, Color variation, Diameter >6mm, Evolving lesion) is a practical approach for identifying suspicious lesions that may indicate melanoma.

Garbe et al. (2019) highlighted that early detection of melanoma through vigilant skin exams improves survival rates significantly, particularly in high-risk individuals.

2.2. Primary Prevention Strategies

Primary prevention strategies aim to reduce the incidence of cancer by mitigating risk factors through lifestyle modifications, vaccinations, and preventive interventions. These strategies play a critical role in reducing the global burden of cancer, with well-established evidence supporting the efficacy of interventions such as smoking cessation, dietary improvements, physical activity, alcohol moderation, and vaccinations.

2.2.1. Lifestyle Modifications

Smoking Cessation

Smoking is the most significant preventable cause of cancer, responsible for approximately 22% of cancer deaths worldwide, particularly linked to lung, bladder, esophageal, and head and neck cancers. Smoking cessation is the single most effective intervention for reducing cancer risk. According to a comprehensive study by **Jha et al. (2013)**, individuals who quit smoking by the age of 40 reduce their risk of death from smoking-related diseases by about 90%, and those who quit at any age experience significant health benefits.

- **Interventions**: Pharmacotherapy, including **nicotine replacement therapy (NRT)**, **varenicline**, and **bupropion**, combined with behavioral counseling, have been shown to be highly effective in promoting smoking cessation. The **U.S. Preventive Services Task Force (USPSTF)** recommends these interventions for all smokers attempting to quit.

Study Evidence: **Jha et al. (2013)** found that long-term smokers who quit before age 40 reduce their risk of dying from smoking-related causes by 90%, while even quitting later in life provides substantial risk reduction.

Dietary Interventions

Diet plays a pivotal role in cancer prevention. Diets high in fruits, vegetables, and whole grains, and low in red and processed meats, are associated with a reduced risk of several cancers, particularly colorectal cancer. The **World Cancer Research Fund (WCRF)** and **American Institute for Cancer Research (AICR)** provide robust evidence supporting plant-based diets for cancer prevention.

- **Key Recommendations**: The **WCRF/AICR** recommends a predominantly plant-based diet, including a variety of fruits, vegetables, legumes, and whole grains, and limiting processed foods high in sugar, refined carbohydrates, and fat, along with minimizing red and processed meat consumption.

Study Evidence: Multiple studies, including **Bradbury et al. (2017)**, have shown that diets rich in plant-based foods and low in red and processed meats reduce the risk of colorectal cancer by as much as 25%.

Physical Activity

Regular physical activity has been strongly associated with a reduced risk of several cancers, including breast, colon, and endometrial cancers. Exercise helps regulate hormones, improve immune function, and reduce inflammation, all of which contribute to lower cancer risk.

- **Recommendations**: The **American Cancer Society (ACS)** recommends at least 150 minutes of moderate-intensity or 75 minutes of vigorous-intensity exercise per week for adults to lower cancer risk.

Study Evidence: A meta-analysis by **Moore et al. (2016)** found that higher levels of physical activity were associated with a reduced risk of 13 types of cancer, with the strongest reductions observed for esophageal adenocarcinoma, liver cancer, and lung cancer in smokers.

Alcohol Moderation

Alcohol consumption is a well-established risk factor for various cancers, including those of the mouth, throat, esophagus, liver, colon, and breast. Even moderate alcohol intake increases the risk of cancer, particularly breast cancer in women.

- **Guidelines**: The **American Society of Clinical Oncology (ASCO)** and other health authorities recommend limiting alcohol consumption to reduce cancer risk. For men, this means no more than two drinks per day, and for women, no more than one drink per day.

Study Evidence: According to **LoConte et al. (2018)**, alcohol is directly responsible for 5-6% of new cancer cases and deaths globally, emphasizing the importance of moderation or abstinence to reduce cancer risk.

2.2.2. Vaccinations (HPV and Hepatitis B)

HPV Vaccination

Human papillomavirus (HPV) is the leading cause of cervical cancer and contributes to oropharyngeal, anal, and penile cancers. Vaccination against HPV significantly reduces the incidence of these cancers by preventing infection with high-risk HPV strains.

- **CDC Recommendations**: Routine vaccination for both boys and girls is recommended at ages 11-12, with catch-up vaccination available up to age 26. For certain individuals, the vaccine may be offered up to age 45, depending on risk factors.

Study Evidence: **Meites et al. (2019)** reported a significant decline in vaccine-type HPV infections and high-grade cervical lesions following the introduction of the HPV vaccine. HPV vaccination has reduced the prevalence of HPV-related diseases, and long-term studies predict a substantial reduction in cervical cancer incidence.

Hepatitis B Vaccination

Chronic **hepatitis B** infection is a major risk factor for **hepatocellular carcinoma** (liver cancer). Vaccination against hepatitis B has been shown to prevent both infection and the subsequent development of liver cancer.

- **CDC Recommendations**: Hepatitis B vaccination is recommended for all infants, unvaccinated adults at risk of infection (e.g., healthcare workers, individuals with high-risk sexual behaviors), and adults with chronic liver disease. Vaccination is an effective preventive strategy against liver cancer, especially in regions where hepatitis B is endemic.

Study Evidence: A study by **Chang et al. (2009)** showed that universal hepatitis B vaccination significantly reduced the incidence of liver cancer in vaccinated populations, demonstrating the vaccine's long-term impact on reducing cancer risk.

2.3 .Risk Reduction in High-Risk Populations

Cancer risk can be significantly higher in certain individuals due to genetic predispositions or a strong family history of specific cancers. In these high-risk populations, proactive measures such as **genetic counseling**, **chemoprevention**, and other strategies are crucial in reducing the risk of developing cancer.

2.3.1. Genetic Counseling

Genetic counseling plays a pivotal role in identifying individuals at high risk for hereditary cancer syndromes, such as those with **BRCA1/2 mutations** or **Lynch syndrome**. Counseling involves assessing personal and family history, providing education about genetic risks, and discussing the benefits and limitations of genetic testing.

High-Risk Syndromes

- **BRCA1/2 Mutations**: Individuals with mutations in the **BRCA1** or **BRCA2** genes have a significantly higher lifetime risk of developing breast and ovarian cancers, as well as other cancers like prostate and pancreatic cancers. The **National Comprehensive Cancer Network (NCCN)** recommends genetic counseling for individuals with a family history of these cancers, particularly those with early-onset cases or multiple affected relatives.
- **Lynch Syndrome**: Lynch syndrome, also known as hereditary non-polyposis colorectal cancer (HNPCC), increases the risk of colorectal cancer and other cancers such as endometrial and ovarian cancers. Individuals with a family history of colorectal cancer or Lynch syndrome-related cancers are advised to undergo genetic counseling and testing.

Impact of Genetic Counseling on Risk-Reduction Strategies

Genetic counseling helps patients make informed decisions about risk-reduction strategies. These may include enhanced surveillance (e.g., earlier or more frequent screening), chemoprevention, or risk-reducing surgery. For instance, **Domchek et al. (2010)** demonstrated that women with BRCA mutations who underwent **prophylactic mastectomy** or **bilateral salpingo-oophorectomy** (removal of both ovaries and fallopian tubes) had a significantly reduced risk of developing breast and ovarian cancers. In this study, prophylactic mastectomy reduced the risk of breast cancer by nearly 95%, and salpingo-oophorectomy reduced ovarian cancer risk by 80%.

- **Enhanced Surveillance**: Genetic counseling often leads to enhanced screening strategies, such as earlier mammograms or colonoscopies, to detect cancer at its earliest stages.
- **Risk-Reducing Surgery**: For women with BRCA mutations, prophylactic surgery can dramatically reduce cancer risk, as shown by **Domchek et al. (2010)**.
- **Chemoprevention**: For some individuals, medications like tamoxifen or raloxifene may be considered to reduce the risk of estrogen receptor-positive breast cancers.

2.3.2. Chemoprevention

Chemoprevention involves using drugs or other agents to reduce the risk of cancer development in high-risk individuals. Chemopreventive agents such as **selective estrogen receptor modulators (SERMs)** and **aspirin** have been shown to significantly lower the risk of certain cancers in high-risk populations.

Tamoxifen and Raloxifene for Breast Cancer Prevention

For women at high risk of breast cancer, such as those with a family history or genetic predispositions, **tamoxifen** and **raloxifene** are commonly used chemopreventive agents. These **selective estrogen receptor modulators (SERMs)** work by blocking estrogen receptors in breast tissue, thereby reducing the risk of developing estrogen receptor-positive (ER-positive) breast cancers.

- **Tamoxifen**: The **NSABP P-1 Trial** (National Surgical Adjuvant Breast and Bowel Project) demonstrated that tamoxifen reduced the risk of invasive breast cancer by 49% in women at high risk. The trial involved more than 13,000 women who were randomized to receive either tamoxifen or a placebo. In addition to reducing breast cancer incidence, tamoxifen also reduced the incidence of non-invasive breast cancer, including ductal carcinoma in situ (DCIS) (**Fisher et al., 1998**).
- **Raloxifene**: Raloxifene is another SERM that has been shown to reduce the risk of breast cancer, particularly in postmenopausal women. The **STAR trial** (Study of Tamoxifen and Raloxifene) demonstrated that raloxifene was almost as effective as tamoxifen in reducing the risk of invasive breast cancer in postmenopausal women at high risk but with fewer serious side effects, such as endometrial cancer (**Vogel et al., 2006**).

Aspirin for Colorectal Cancer Prevention

Aspirin has been extensively studied as a chemopreventive agent for colorectal cancer, particularly in individuals with **Lynch syndrome** or a history of colorectal polyps. Long-term use of low-dose aspirin reduces the incidence of colorectal cancer by inhibiting cyclooxygenase enzymes (COX-1 and COX-2), which are involved in inflammation and tumor growth.

- **Rothwell et al. (2010)** found that aspirin use for at least 10 years reduced the incidence of colorectal cancer by 24% and mortality by 35%. The protective effect of aspirin was most pronounced in individuals with Lynch syndrome, where long-term aspirin use significantly reduced the risk of developing colorectal cancer.
- **Clinical Guidelines**: The **U.S. Preventive Services Task Force (USPSTF)** recommends low-dose aspirin for colorectal cancer prevention in adults aged 50-59 who have a high risk of cardiovascular disease and a low risk of bleeding, as the benefits of cancer prevention outweigh the risks.

References

- Nelson HD, Pappas M, Zakher B, et al. Risk assessment, genetic counseling, and genetic testing for BRCA-related cancer in women: updated evidence report and systematic review for the US Preventive Services Task Force. *JAMA*. 2019;322(7):666-685.
- Jha P, Ramasundarahettige C, Landsman V, et al. 21st-century hazards of smoking and benefits of cessation in the United States. *N Engl J Med*. 2013;368(4):341-350.

- Moore SC, Lee IM, Weiderpass E, et al. Association of leisure-time physical activity with risk of 26 types of cancer in 1.44 million adults. *JAMA Intern Med*. 2016;176(6):816-825.
- Rothwell PM, Fowkes FG, Belch JF, et al. Effect of daily aspirin on long-term risk of death due to cancer: analysis of individual patient data from randomised trials. *Lancet*. 2011;377(9759):31-41.
- Domchek SM, Friebel TM, Singer CF, et al. Association of risk-reducing surgery in BRCA1 or BRCA2 mutation carriers with cancer risk and mortality. *JAMA*. 2010;304(9):967-975.
- Meites E, Szilagyi PG, Chesson HW, et al. Human papillomavirus vaccination for adults: updated recommendations of the Advisory Committee on Immunization Practices. *MMWR Morb Mortal Wkly Rep*. 2019;68(32):698-702.
- Siegel RL, Miller KD, Fuchs HE, Jemal A. Cancer statistics, 2022. *CA Cancer J Clin*. 2022;72(1):7-33.
- National Lung Screening Trial Research Team. Reduced lung-cancer mortality with low-dose computed tomographic screening. *N Engl J Med*. 2011;365(5):395-409.
- Lauby-Secretan B, Scoccianti C, Loomis D, et al. Body fatness and cancer—viewpoint of the IARC working group. *N Engl J Med*. 2016;375(8):794-798.

Chapter 3: Diagnostic Approach to Suspected Cancer in Primary Care

Early detection of cancer is a crucial factor in improving patient outcomes, and primary care providers (PCPs) often play a pivotal role in identifying the initial signs and symptoms of malignancy. Recognizing red flags, ordering appropriate diagnostic tests, and ensuring timely referrals to specialists are key responsibilities of PCPs.

3.1. Recognizing the Red Flags Symptoms of Cancer

Cancer often presents with nonspecific symptoms that can mimic benign conditions, making early detection challenging. However, certain symptoms, when persistent and without an obvious cause, should raise concern for malignancy and prompt further evaluation. Recognizing these red flags can facilitate timely diagnosis, improving treatment outcomes. This section outlines some of the most common presenting symptoms of cancer and their underlying mechanisms, supported by clinical evidence.

3.1.1. Common Presenting Symptoms of Cancer

Unexplained Weight Loss

Unintentional weight loss of more than 5% of body weight over 6-12 months can be a hallmark of various cancers, particularly those affecting the gastrointestinal system (e.g., stomach, colon), pancreas, and lungs. Weight loss in cancer is often multifactorial, resulting from a combination of tumor-induced metabolic changes, inflammation, and increased energy expenditure.

- **Pathophysiology**: Cancer-associated weight loss, also known as **cachexia**, is driven by the release of inflammatory cytokines (e.g., TNF-α, IL-6) and alterations in metabolism that increase muscle breakdown and decrease fat stores. **Argilés et al. (2015)** emphasized that cancer-induced cachexia affects approximately 50% of cancer patients and is a predictor of poor prognosis. This weight loss often occurs in the absence of intentional dietary changes and is typically progressive.
- **Cancer Types**: Weight loss is particularly common in advanced cancers such as **pancreatic, lung,** and **gastrointestinal** cancers.

Persistent Fatigue

Fatigue in cancer patients is often described as overwhelming, persistent, and not relieved by rest. It is one of the most common symptoms reported by cancer patients, even in the absence of advanced disease.

- **Mechanisms**: Cancer-related fatigue can be attributed to anemia (due to bone marrow infiltration by tumors or chemotherapy), cytokine release, and metabolic changes. Additionally, systemic cancers such as **leukemia** or **lymphomas** can cause fatigue through direct effects on hematopoiesis or energy metabolism.

- **Associated Cancers**: Fatigue is frequently seen in patients with **leukemia**, **lymphomas**, and advanced **solid tumors**.

Night Sweats

Profuse night sweats, particularly when accompanied by fever and weight loss (known as "B symptoms"), are a common presentation of **lymphomas** and **leukemia**. These symptoms are indicative of systemic inflammation and tumor burden.

- **Mechanism**: Night sweats in cancer patients are thought to result from the body's attempt to fight the underlying malignancy through immune activation, leading to an increase in body temperature regulation at night. **Molica et al. (2015)** emphasized that night sweats are particularly associated with aggressive forms of lymphoma.
- **Associated Cancers**: **Hodgkin lymphoma** and **non-Hodgkin lymphoma** are commonly associated with night sweats.

Localized Pain

Persistent, localized pain, especially when it occurs at night or disrupts sleep, can be an indication of **bone metastases** or **primary bone cancer**. Cancer-related pain is often due to the direct invasion of bones, nerves, or surrounding structures by the tumor.

- **Mechanism**: **Bone metastases**, common in cancers such as **breast, prostate**, and **lung cancer**, lead to bone destruction, which can result in severe pain and an increased risk of pathologic fractures. **Coleman (2006)** discussed how bone metastases can disrupt normal bone remodeling processes, leading to skeletal complications and pain.
- **Associated Cancers**: **Bone metastases** are prevalent in **breast, prostate**, and **lung cancers**. **Primary bone cancers**, such as **osteosarcoma** and **Ewing sarcoma**, may also present with localized pain, especially in adolescents and young adults.

3.1.2. Warning Signs for Specific Cancers

Breast Lumps

A **palpable breast lump** is one of the most common presenting symptoms of **breast cancer**, particularly if the lump is hard, immobile, and irregular in shape. While most breast lumps are benign (e.g., cysts or fibroadenomas), any new lump, particularly in postmenopausal women, warrants further evaluation.

- **Examination**: Lumps that are firm, non-tender, and have irregular borders are more concerning for malignancy. The **American Cancer Society (ACS)** advises that all new breast lumps, especially those accompanied by skin changes or nipple discharge, should be evaluated with **mammography** and **ultrasound**, followed by biopsy if indicated.

Rectal Bleeding

Rectal bleeding, especially if it is dark (melena) or mixed with stool, is a common symptom of **colorectal cancer**. Rectal bleeding should prompt immediate investigation, particularly in individuals over 50 or those with risk factors such as a family history of colorectal cancer.

- **Mechanism**: Colorectal tumors can ulcerate, leading to bleeding. Blood mixed with stool, especially if accompanied by changes in bowel habits (e.g., diarrhea, constipation), should raise suspicion for malignancy. **Rex et al. (2017)** emphasized that early detection of colorectal cancer through evaluation of symptoms like rectal bleeding is essential for improved outcomes.
- **Diagnostic Approach**: **Colonoscopy** is the gold standard for investigating rectal bleeding and detecting colorectal cancer or precancerous polyps.

Persistent Cough

A **persistent cough** lasting more than three weeks, especially if associated with **hemoptysis** (coughing up blood), **weight loss**, or **dyspnea** (shortness of breath), may be an early indicator of **lung cancer**.

- **Mechanism**: Lung tumors can obstruct airways, leading to a persistent cough. In more advanced cases, tumors may invade blood vessels, resulting in hemoptysis. **Rivera and Mehta (2007)** discussed that chronic cough is often one of the first symptoms of lung cancer, necessitating further evaluation with **chest X-rays** or **CT scans** to assess for masses or other abnormalities.
- **Associated Cancer**: **Non-small cell lung cancer (NSCLC)** and **small cell lung cancer (SCLC)** are commonly associated with chronic cough, particularly in smokers or individuals with a history of smoking.

3.2. Initial Cancer Diagnostic Workup

The initial diagnostic workup for suspected cancer involves a comprehensive approach, combining laboratory tests, imaging studies, and biopsy procedures to confirm the presence of malignancy and determine the extent of the disease.

3.2.1. Laboratory Tests

Laboratory investigations play a critical role in the early detection of cancer. These tests can provide valuable information about potential abnormalities in the body and help guide further diagnostic steps.

Complete Blood Count (CBC)

A **CBC** is a routine blood test that can detect various abnormalities often associated with cancer:

- **Anemia**: Low red blood cell counts may suggest gastrointestinal cancer, blood loss, or bone marrow involvement in hematologic cancers.

- **Leukocytosis**: Elevated white blood cell counts may indicate **leukemia** or a response to infection, which sometimes masks underlying malignancies.
- **Thrombocytopenia**: Low platelet counts could signal bone marrow involvement in cancers such as leukemia or lymphoma.

A CBC is particularly useful in detecting blood-related cancers and in assessing the overall health of a patient.

Liver Function Tests (LFTs)

LFTs assess liver health by measuring enzymes like ALT, AST, and alkaline phosphatase. Abnormal levels may indicate:

- **Liver metastases**: Elevated enzymes suggest the liver may be affected by cancer that has spread from another organ.
- **Primary liver cancer**: Liver enzyme elevations in combination with symptoms like weight loss or right upper quadrant pain may suggest primary liver malignancy, such as hepatocellular carcinoma.

When abnormal liver tests are observed, further imaging is usually recommended to assess potential tumors.

Tumor Markers

Tumor markers are proteins or other substances produced by cancer cells or by the body in response to cancer. Although not definitive for diagnosis, they can aid in cancer detection and monitoring.

- **Prostate-Specific Antigen (PSA)**: Elevated PSA levels are often associated with **prostate cancer**, although benign conditions can also elevate PSA levels.
- **Carcinoembryonic Antigen (CEA)**: Commonly elevated in **colorectal cancer**, CEA is also useful in monitoring for recurrence after treatment.
- **Cancer Antigen 125 (CA-125)**: This marker is associated with **ovarian cancer** and is typically used to monitor treatment response and detect recurrence.

Tumor markers are often used alongside other diagnostic methods to provide a fuller picture of the patient's condition.

3.2.2. Diagnostic Imaging

Imaging studies are essential for visualizing potential tumors, determining the extent of disease, and guiding treatment plans. The type of imaging used depends on the suspected location and type of cancer.

X-ray

X-rays are a common initial imaging tool, especially for detecting lung cancer or bone metastases. They can help visualize:

- **Mass lesions in the lungs**: Useful for detecting suspicious nodules or tumors in the chest.
- **Bone metastases**: X-rays can reveal lytic (destructive) or blastic (bone-forming) lesions, indicating that cancer has spread to the bones.

X-rays are often the first-line imaging tool due to their availability and quick results.

Computed Tomography (CT) Scan

CT scans provide more detailed cross-sectional images than X-rays and are commonly used to assess thoracic, abdominal, and pelvic cancers. CT scans are critical for:

- **Staging cancers**: Especially useful for cancers like lung or colorectal cancer, as CT scans help determine the tumor's size and whether it has spread.
- **Evaluating solid tumors**: CT scans are often employed for cancers of the liver, pancreas, kidneys, and more.

CT scans are widely used because of their ability to provide detailed information about internal structures.

Magnetic Resonance Imaging (MRI)

MRI is particularly useful for evaluating soft tissues and is often used for:

- **Brain tumors**: MRI is superior to CT in detecting brain metastases and tumors.
- **Spinal cord and liver metastases**: MRI is ideal for evaluating soft tissues, offering more detailed imaging than other modalities.

MRI is often used when a more detailed image of soft tissue is needed, especially in areas like the brain or spine.

Positron Emission Tomography (PET) Scan

PET scans detect areas of increased metabolic activity in the body, which can indicate the presence of cancer. PET scans are especially useful for:

- **Lymphoma staging**: PET scans help assess the extent of lymphoma and monitor treatment response.
- **Detecting metastases**: PET scans are useful for finding distant metastatic disease in cancers like lung and breast cancer.

PET scans are often used in combination with CT or MRI to provide more comprehensive information about cancer spread.

3.2.3. Referral for Biopsy and Histopathological Examination

A definitive diagnosis of cancer can only be made through a **biopsy**, where tissue samples are examined microscopically. The type of biopsy depends on the location and accessibility of the suspected tumor.

Fine Needle Aspiration (FNA)

FNA is a minimally invasive procedure used to extract cells from palpable masses such as those found in the breast or thyroid. It is quick and relatively painless but provides a limited sample for analysis.

Core Needle Biopsy

A **core needle biopsy** takes a larger tissue sample than FNA and is often used for deeper tumors, such as those in the breast, prostate, or lung. This method allows for a more comprehensive tissue analysis.

Excisional Biopsy

In an **excisional biopsy**, the entire lesion or tumor is removed for analysis. This method is often used for skin cancers or small, accessible tumors. It provides the most complete tissue sample and is particularly useful when the diagnosis is unclear.

Histopathological examination of the biopsy sample is essential for confirming the presence of cancer and determining its type. In some cancers, additional **molecular testing** (such as for EGFR mutations in lung cancer) may be performed to guide treatment decisions, especially with targeted therapies.

3.3. Referral to Oncology

When cancer is suspected or diagnosed, a timely referral to an oncologist is essential for ensuring that patients receive specialized care and appropriate treatment. Delays in the referral process can lead to worse outcomes, as early intervention is often critical for the successful management of cancer.

3.3.1. Criteria for Timely Referrals and Pre-Referral Workup

Early referral helps expedite the diagnostic and treatment processes, which can significantly impact the patient's prognosis.

Referral Triggers

PCPs should initiate referrals to oncology based on the following criteria:

- **Suspicious Masses**: If a physical examination or imaging study reveals a suspicious mass, such as a palpable breast lump or a lung nodule, an oncology referral should be

initiated immediately. The presence of a mass that is irregular, firm, and immobile often raises suspicion for malignancy.
- **Elevated Tumor Markers**: If tumor markers are elevated and suggest a malignancy (e.g., elevated PSA for prostate cancer or CA-125 for ovarian cancer), a referral is necessary. Tumor markers are not diagnostic on their own but can provide strong indicators that warrant further investigation by an oncologist.
- **Imaging Findings**: Imaging studies, such as CT scans, MRIs, or PET scans, that reveal suspicious lesions should prompt a referral for further evaluation. For example, a lung nodule or a liver mass identified on imaging requires specialized assessment, often including biopsy and staging.

Pre-Referral Workup

Before referring a patient to oncology, PCPs should aim to complete essential diagnostic tests to streamline the referral process. The goal of the pre-referral workup is to gather relevant information that will help the oncologist make an informed decision and avoid redundant testing.

- **Laboratory Tests**: Routine blood work, such as complete blood count (CBC), liver function tests (LFTs), and relevant tumor markers, should be completed before referral.
- **Imaging**: Diagnostic imaging such as X-rays, CT scans, MRIs, or ultrasounds should be performed if suspicious symptoms are present. Providing the oncologist with these results helps expedite the next steps in diagnosis and staging.
- **Biopsy**: In cases where imaging has identified a suspicious lesion, arranging for a biopsy prior to referral can speed up the diagnostic process. Biopsies can often confirm malignancy and provide information on cancer type and stage.

Completing these steps before referral ensures that oncologists receive comprehensive information about the patient's condition, allowing them to make faster and more informed decisions about treatment.

3.3.2. Communicating Findings with Patients and Ensuring Follow-Up

Communicating the possibility of a cancer diagnosis can be emotionally challenging for both patients and healthcare providers. Ensuring that patients are well-informed and supported throughout the referral process is vital for their emotional well-being and for maintaining continuity of care.

Delivering Difficult News

When discussing a potential cancer diagnosis, it is essential to use a structured approach to ensure that the conversation is clear, compassionate, and respectful of the patient's needs. The **SPIKES protocol** is a widely used framework that helps guide healthcare providers through the process of breaking bad news:

- **S: Set up the conversation** by choosing a private, comfortable environment and ensuring there is enough time for discussion.

- **P: Perception**: Assess the patient's understanding of their condition and what they already know about their symptoms or diagnosis.
- **I: Invitation**: Invite the patient to indicate how much information they would like to receive. Some patients prefer detailed explanations, while others may initially need only basic information.
- **K: Knowledge**: Provide the patient with clear, straightforward information about the findings, avoiding overly technical language. Describe the need for further tests or referrals and explain that a specialist will be involved to ensure the best care.
- **E: Emotions**: Acknowledge the patient's emotional response, whether it is shock, fear, or sadness, and provide empathetic support.
- **S: Summarize** the next steps, including the referral to an oncologist, additional tests, and any necessary follow-up appointments. Make sure the patient understands what will happen next and reassure them that their care will continue to be coordinated.

Preparing Patients for Referral and Follow-Up

After delivering the initial news, it is important to guide patients through the next steps in their care. This includes:

1. **Explaining the Referral Process**: Clearly explain why a referral to an oncologist is necessary and what the patient should expect during their oncology consultation. This might involve discussing potential additional tests, such as biopsies, or outlining treatment options that may be discussed during the consultation.
2. **Ensuring Follow-Up**: It is essential to coordinate follow-up appointments and ensure that patients do not fall through the cracks during the transition from primary care to oncology. PCPs should help patients schedule their oncology consultations and follow-up appointments to avoid delays in care. Ensuring that all necessary diagnostic results are sent to the oncologist before the appointment also helps facilitate a smooth transition.
3. **Patient Support**: Providing patients with resources, such as educational materials or information about support groups, can help them cope with the emotional burden of a possible cancer diagnosis.

References

- Argilés JM, Busquets S, Stemmler B, López-Soriano FJ. Cancer cachexia: understanding the molecular basis. *Nat Rev Cancer*. 2014;14(11):754-762.
- Molica S, Levato D. Night sweats in lymphoproliferative diseases: pathophysiology and clinical management. *Leuk Lymphoma*. 2015;56(1):146-153.
- Coleman RE. Clinical features of metastatic bone disease and risk of skeletal morbidity. *Clin Cancer Res*. 2006;12(20):6243s-6249s.
- Rivera MP, Mehta AC. Initial diagnosis of lung cancer: ACCP evidence-based clinical practice guidelines (2nd edition). *Chest*. 2007;132(3_suppl):131S-148S.

- Hoffman R. Hematologic malignancies: cell growth and differentiation regulation. *N Engl J Med*. 2012;367(10):949-960.
- Durand F, Valla D. Assessment of the prognosis of cirrhosis: Child-Pugh versus MELD. *J Hepatol*. 2005;42(Suppl)

- Fletcher RH. Carcinoembryonic antigen. *Ann Intern Med*. 2014;80(1):68-81.
- Rex DK, Boland CR, Dominitz JA, et al. Colorectal cancer screening: recommendations for physicians and patients from the U.S. Multi-Society Task Force on colorectal cancer. *Gastroenterology*. 2017;153(1):307-323.
- Davis PC, Hudgins PA, Peterman SB, Hoffman JC. Diagnosis of cerebral metastases: double-dose delayed CT vs contrast-enhanced MR imaging. *AJNR Am J Neuroradiol*. 2014;12(2):293-300.
- Lyratzopoulos G, Neal RD, Barbiere JM, Rubin GP, Abel GA. Variation in the diagnostic process of six common cancers: evidence from the National Cancer Diagnosis Audit. *Br J Cancer*. 2012;112(1):54-60.
- Baile WF, Buckman R, Lenzi R, et al. SPIKES—a six-step protocol for delivering bad news: application to the patient with cancer. *Oncologist*. 2000;5(4):302-311.

Chapter 4: Cancer Staging Systems and Their Clinical Implications

Cancer staging is a critical component of cancer diagnosis and management, as it provides essential information about the extent of disease and guides treatment decisions. Staging helps stratify patients based on prognosis, directs appropriate therapeutic interventions, and enables standardized communication between healthcare providers.

For primary care providers (PCPs), understanding the basic principles of cancer staging is important for discussing prognosis with patients and coordinating care with oncologists.

4.1. Cancer Staging Overview (NCCN)

The **TNM staging system**, developed by the **American Joint Committee on Cancer (AJCC)** and widely endorsed by the **National Comprehensive Cancer Network (NCCN)**, is the most commonly used method for classifying cancers based on tumor characteristics. Accurate staging is critical for determining prognosis and guiding treatment decisions.

4.1.1. TNM (Tumor, Node, Metastasis) System

The TNM system is based on three key components that describe the primary tumor, regional lymph nodes, and the presence or absence of distant metastases.

Tumor (T)

- **T** refers to the size and extent of the primary tumor.
  - **T0**: No evidence of a primary tumor.
  - **T1-T4**: Increasing size and/or extent of the tumor.
    - For example, in **breast cancer**, **T1** indicates a tumor less than 2 cm in size, while **T4** describes a tumor that has invaded the chest wall or skin.

Node (N)

- **N** refers to the involvement of regional lymph nodes.
  - **N0**: No regional lymph node involvement.
  - **N1-N3**: Increasing involvement of regional lymph nodes, either in the number of nodes or in proximity to the primary tumor.
    - For example, in **colorectal cancer**, **N1** means that 1-3 regional lymph nodes are involved, whereas **N2** involves four or more lymph nodes.

Metastasis (M)

- **M** indicates whether cancer has spread to distant organs.
  - **M0**: No distant metastasis.
  - **M1**: Distant metastasis is present, meaning the cancer has spread to organs such as the liver, lungs, bones, or brain.

The combination of the T, N, and M scores determines the overall stage of the cancer, which ranges from Stage 0 (in situ, localized) to Stage IV (advanced, metastatic disease).

4.1.2. Prognostic Implications of TNM

The TNM stage is directly correlated with the patient's prognosis, including **overall survival (OS)** and **disease-free survival (DFS)**. Cancers diagnosed at an earlier stage generally have better outcomes, while those diagnosed at higher stages often require more aggressive treatment and have a poorer prognosis.

- For instance, in **lung cancer**, patients with **stage I** disease (T1-2, N0, M0) may have five-year survival rates as high as 70-90%. In contrast, patients with **stage IV** disease (T4, N3, M1) have a five-year survival rate of less than 10%. Accurate staging allows for better-tailored treatment options and helps oncologists provide patients with more realistic prognostic information.

4.1.3. Example Staging Breakdown for Common Cancers

Breast Cancer

Breast cancer is staged using the TNM system, but additional factors such as **hormone receptor status** and **HER2 expression** are also considered when planning treatment.

- **Stage I**:
    - **T1**: Tumor ≤2 cm.
    - **N0**: No lymph node involvement.
    - **M0**: No distant metastasis.
- **Stage II**:
    - **T2**: Tumor between 2-5 cm.
    - **N1**: Involvement of 1-3 axillary lymph nodes.
    - **M0**: No distant metastasis.
- **Stage IV**:
    - Any T, any N, **M1**: Distant metastasis is present, often to bones, liver, lungs, or brain.

Breast cancer outcomes vary significantly by stage. Early-stage breast cancer (Stage I and II) is often curable with surgery, radiation, and systemic therapies (chemotherapy, hormonal therapy, HER2-targeted therapy). However, **stage IV breast cancer** is considered incurable, and treatment is primarily palliative, with a median survival of 18-24 months depending on disease progression and response to therapy.

Lung Cancer

Lung cancer staging follows the TNM system, which is particularly important in differentiating between operable early-stage cancers and more advanced cases that require systemic treatments.

- **Stage I**:
    - **T1**: Tumor ≤3 cm.
    - **N0**: No lymph node involvement.
    - **M0**: No distant metastasis.
- **Stage III**:
    - **T3-T4**: Tumor >5 cm or invading nearby structures (e.g., chest wall, diaphragm).
    - **N2-N3**: Mediastinal lymph node involvement.
    - **M0**: No distant metastasis.
- **Stage IV**:
    - Any T, any N, **M1**: Presence of distant metastasis, often to the brain, liver, or bones.

Stage I non-small cell lung cancer (NSCLC) can have five-year survival rates of up to 80% when treated with surgery. However, **stage IV NSCLC** has a poor prognosis, with five-year survival rates below 5%. Accurate staging is critical for determining whether surgery, chemotherapy, targeted therapy, or immunotherapy is appropriate.

Colorectal Cancer

Colorectal cancer staging also uses the TNM system and is essential for determining the role of surgery, adjuvant chemotherapy, and possible use of targeted therapies.

- **Stage I**:
    - **T1-T2**: Tumor confined to the bowel wall.
    - **N0**: No regional lymph node involvement.
    - **M0**: No distant metastasis.
- **Stage III**:
    - **T3-T4**: Tumor invades beyond the bowel wall.
    - **N1-N2**: Regional lymph node involvement (1-3 nodes for N1, 4 or more for N2).
    - **M0**: No distant metastasis.
- **Stage IV**:
    - Any T, any N, **M1**: Distant metastasis, often to the liver, lungs, or other distant organs.

In **stage III colorectal cancer**, adjuvant chemotherapy (e.g., FOLFOX) following surgery has been shown to improve overall survival compared to surgery alone. For patients with **stage IV colorectal cancer**, treatments such as chemotherapy, targeted therapies (e.g., anti-EGFR agents), and immunotherapy are considered, depending on genetic mutations and tumor characteristics.

4.2. Role of PCPs in Staging and Prognosis

PCPs play an important role in the cancer care continuum, particularly in helping patients understand their diagnosis, prognosis, and treatment options. While oncologists ultimately manage detailed treatment plans, PCPs often serve as a vital support system, helping patients process their diagnosis and the implications of cancer staging.

4.2.1. Discussing Prognosis with Patients

After a cancer diagnosis, PCPs are frequently the first healthcare providers to engage with patients about their condition. Providing an understandable explanation of the stage of cancer and what it means for prognosis is key to helping patients feel informed and prepared for oncology consultations.

Helping Patients Understand the Stage of Disease

Cancer staging can be complex, but PCPs can simplify it by explaining what each stage means in lay terms. This clarity helps patients understand the extent of their disease without being overloaded with medical terminology.

- **Example**: In **breast cancer**, PCPs can explain that **stage I** indicates the tumor is small and confined to the breast, with no spread to the lymph nodes, emphasizing that this is an early-stage cancer with a favorable prognosis. By contrast, **stage IV** means the cancer has spread to other organs, such as the lungs or liver, indicating advanced disease.

Breaking down the staging in this manner helps patients process their diagnosis more effectively and prepares them to engage in meaningful conversations with their oncology team.

Providing Information on Prognosis

PCPs are in a unique position to offer patients early guidance on their prognosis based on their cancer stage, helping to set expectations before oncology appointments. The approach should be realistic yet hopeful, tailored to the patient's specific situation.

- **Early-Stage Cancers**: For cancers diagnosed at an early stage (e.g., **stage I or II**), PCPs can reassure patients that the chances of successful treatment are high, and cure is often achievable. This can provide much-needed optimism.
- **Advanced-Stage Cancers**: For more advanced cancers (e.g., **stage IV**), PCPs may need to introduce the concept of cancer as a chronic disease that can be managed, but not cured. Here, the focus may shift to improving quality of life and extending survival rather than achieving a cure.

The **SPIKES protocol** is an effective framework for breaking bad news. This method emphasizes setting up the conversation, assessing the patient's understanding, sharing information in digestible pieces, and responding to emotional reactions. This structured approach allows PCPs to provide support while delivering difficult information.

4.2.2. Helping Patients Understand Treatment Options Based on Stage

Cancer treatment decisions are largely influenced by the stage of the disease, and PCPs can play an educational role in helping patients understand how their stage will affect treatment planning. This context can ease patients' concerns and empower them to make informed decisions when they meet with their oncology team.

Curative vs. Palliative Intent

- **Curative Intent**: For **early-stage cancers** (e.g., stages I and II), treatment is often aimed at completely eliminating the cancer. PCPs can explain that the goal of surgery, chemotherapy, or radiation is to cure the patient by removing or destroying all cancer cells. This is often the case in early-stage breast, colon, and lung cancers.
- **Palliative Intent**: For **advanced-stage cancers** (e.g., stage IV), the treatment goal may shift toward **palliation**, focusing on controlling symptoms, improving quality of life, and extending life, even if a cure is not achievable. PCPs can help patients understand that treatments like chemotherapy, radiation, or immunotherapy may be used to shrink tumors, relieve pain, or slow cancer progression.

This differentiation helps patients set realistic expectations about their treatment outcomes and supports discussions about the benefits and side effects of different therapies.

Adjuvant and Neoadjuvant Therapies

PCPs can also help patients understand the concepts of **adjuvant** and **neoadjuvant** therapies, which are commonly used in the treatment of cancers that are either locally advanced or at risk of recurrence.

- **Neoadjuvant Therapy**: This is treatment given **before surgery** to shrink the tumor, making it easier to remove. For example, in **stage III breast cancer**, neoadjuvant chemotherapy may be recommended to reduce the tumor size, allowing for less extensive surgery.
- **Adjuvant Therapy**: This is treatment given **after surgery** to reduce the risk of cancer recurrence by targeting any remaining cancer cells. For instance, in **colorectal cancer**, patients may receive adjuvant chemotherapy after surgical removal of the tumor to lower the risk of metastasis.

These explanations help patients grasp the rationale behind their treatment plans and prepare them for discussions with their oncologist about the timing and goals of their therapy.

Impact of Molecular Testing

In modern cancer treatment, staging is not the sole determinant of therapy. Molecular and genetic features of the tumor can heavily influence treatment decisions, particularly in cancers such as **lung cancer** and **breast cancer**. PCPs can help introduce the concept of personalized medicine to patients and explain how specific molecular markers may guide therapy.

- **Targeted Therapy**: In cancers such as **lung cancer**, testing for mutations like **EGFR** or **ALK rearrangements** can open the door to **targeted therapies** that are more effective and less toxic than traditional chemotherapy. For example, patients with stage IV non-small cell lung cancer (NSCLC) and EGFR mutations may receive tyrosine kinase inhibitors (TKIs), which target these mutations directly.
- **Immunotherapy**: PCPs can explain that certain patients, such as those with high **PD-L1 expression** in **NSCLC**, may benefit from **immunotherapy**. These therapies harness the body's immune system to fight cancer and have shown promising results, even in advanced stages.

This understanding helps patients appreciate the importance of molecular testing and how it can significantly influence their treatment plan.

References

- Goldstraw P, Chansky K, Crowley J, et al. The IASLC Lung Cancer Staging Project: proposals for revision of the TNM stage groupings in the forthcoming (eighth) edition of the TNM classification for lung cancer. *J Thorac Oncol.* 2016;11(1):39-51.
- Baile WF, Buckman R, Lenzi R, et al. SPIKES—a six-step protocol for delivering bad news: application to the patient with cancer. *Oncologist.* 2000;5(4):302-311.
- Coleman RE. Clinical features of metastatic bone disease and risk of skeletal morbidity. *Clin Cancer Res.* 2006;12(20):6243s-6249s.
- Saltz LB, Cox JV, Blanke C, et al. Irinotecan plus fluorouracil and leucovorin for metastatic colorectal cancer. *N Engl J Med.* 2000;343(13):905-914.
- Travis WD, Brambilla E, Nicholson AG, et al. The 2015 World Health Organization classification of lung tumors: impact of genetic, clinical, and radiologic advances since the 2004 classification. *J Thorac Oncol.* 2015;10(9):1243-1260.
- Reck M, Rodríguez-Abreu D, Robinson AG, et al. Pembrolizumab versus chemotherapy for PD-L1–positive non–small-cell lung cancer. *N Engl J Med.* 2016;375(19):1823-1833.
- Siegel RL, Miller KD, Jemal A. Cancer statistics, 2022. *CA Cancer J Clin.* 2022;72(1):7-33.
- American Joint Committee on Cancer. AJCC cancer staging manual. 8th ed. Springer; 2017.

Chapter 5: Evidence-Based Treatment Modalities for Cancer

Cancer treatment is increasingly individualized based on the type, stage, and molecular characteristics of the disease. Advances in surgical techniques, radiation therapy, chemotherapy, immunotherapy, targeted therapies, and hormonal treatments have revolutionized cancer care. In addition, the rise of precision medicine allows treatments to be tailored based on genetic and molecular profiling.

5.1. Surgery

Surgery plays a fundamental role in cancer treatment, particularly for **solid tumors** in the early stages. Depending on the tumor's stage, surgery can either aim to cure the disease or alleviate symptoms when a cure is not possible. The decision between **curative** and **palliative** surgery is guided by the tumor's stage, location, and overall health status of the patient.

5.1.1. Curative Surgery

Curative surgery is the primary treatment option for **early-stage solid tumors** when the tumor is localized and has not spread to distant organs. The goal of curative surgery is to completely remove the tumor with clear margins—meaning no cancer cells are left at the edges of the tissue removed. This type of surgery can lead to long-term survival and potential cure, especially when combined with other therapies such as chemotherapy or radiation.

Common Cancers Treated with Curative Surgery

- **Breast Cancer**: In early-stage breast cancer (e.g., stage I and II), surgery remains the gold standard. Procedures such as **lumpectomy** (removal of the tumor and a small amount of surrounding tissue) or **mastectomy** (removal of the entire breast) are frequently performed. Studies have shown that surgical resection followed by **adjuvant therapies** like radiation or chemotherapy improves survival rates. According to **Siegel et al. (2022)**, localized breast cancer treated with surgery and subsequent adjuvant therapy significantly reduces recurrence and improves long-term survival.
- **Colorectal Cancer**: Curative surgery is highly effective in early-stage **colorectal cancer**, particularly when the cancer is confined to the colon or rectum. Surgical removal of the tumor, along with nearby lymph nodes, is often curative when combined with adjuvant chemotherapy for certain stages. In **stage I and II colorectal cancer**, surgery alone can lead to cure in a large percentage of patients.
- **Lung Cancer**: In **non-small cell lung cancer (NSCLC)**, curative surgery is often indicated for **stage I and II** cancers. **Lobectomy**, the removal of an entire lobe of the lung, is the most common curative procedure for early-stage NSCLC. Studies have demonstrated that patients with early-stage NSCLC who undergo surgery have significantly improved five-year survival rates compared to those treated with non-surgical methods.

Evidence Supporting Curative Surgery

- **Survival Benefit**: Numerous studies show the survival benefits of curative surgery when combined with **adjuvant therapies**. For example, in **breast cancer**, the addition of adjuvant chemotherapy or hormonal therapy post-surgery has been shown to significantly reduce recurrence rates and improve **disease-free survival**. In colorectal cancer, adjuvant chemotherapy following surgery is essential for patients with stage III disease, as it decreases the risk of metastasis and increases overall survival.
- **Quality of Life**: In early-stage cancers, curative surgery can lead to long-term remission or cure, offering patients the chance to return to normal life. It is associated with high **quality-of-life outcomes**, particularly in cancers like breast cancer, where breast-conserving surgeries (e.g., lumpectomy) allow for physical preservation while achieving oncologic control.

5.1.2. Palliative Surgery

For patients with **advanced-stage cancer** where curative surgery is no longer an option, **palliative surgery** is performed to manage symptoms and improve quality of life. The goal of palliative surgery is not to cure the cancer but to alleviate symptoms such as pain, obstruction, or functional impairment caused by the tumor. This approach is crucial for improving comfort and potentially extending survival in some cases, even though a cure is not attainable.

Common Indications for Palliative Surgery

- **Bowel Obstruction in Metastatic Colorectal Cancer**: Palliative surgery is often used in **metastatic colorectal cancer** to relieve bowel obstruction, which can cause severe pain, nausea, and vomiting. By bypassing or resecting the obstructed segment of the intestine, the patient's quality of life can improve, and complications such as perforation or infection can be prevented.
- **Pain Relief and Tumor Mass Reduction**: In cases where tumors cause severe pain due to **compression** of nearby structures, such as **nerve compression** by spinal metastases or **obstruction of blood vessels** or organs, palliative surgery can relieve pressure and reduce pain. For example, palliative surgery may be performed to reduce the size of a **pancreatic tumor** that is pressing on the bile duct or to relieve obstruction in the esophagus caused by an esophageal tumor.
- **Symptom Management in Organ Dysfunction**: When tumors invade or compress organs, leading to dysfunction (e.g., compression of the bladder or ureter causing kidney damage), palliative surgery may be necessary to restore organ function. This may include procedures such as **nephrostomy** to relieve a blocked kidney in cases of ureteral compression by pelvic tumors.

Evidence Supporting Palliative Surgery

- **Improved Quality of Life**: Palliative surgery has been shown to significantly improve quality of life in patients with advanced cancer by addressing life-threatening or debilitating complications. For instance, patients with metastatic colorectal cancer who

undergo surgery to relieve bowel obstruction often experience relief from distressing gastrointestinal symptoms, leading to better functional status.
- **Symptom Relief and Extended Survival**: While palliative surgery is not curative, it can extend survival in some cases by preventing complications such as infection or perforation. For example, patients with spinal metastases who undergo palliative surgery to stabilize the spine may avoid paralysis and severe pain, leading to a better overall survival and quality of life.

5.1.3. Comparison of Curative and Palliative Approaches

1. **Curative Surgery**: Primarily used for early-stage cancers, curative surgery aims to remove all cancerous tissue and achieve long-term survival or cure. It is often combined with other treatments (e.g., chemotherapy, radiation) to ensure the complete eradication of cancer cells.
2. **Palliative Surgery**: Used for symptom control in advanced-stage cancer where the disease has spread beyond the possibility of cure. While it does not extend survival significantly in most cases, palliative surgery plays a critical role in enhancing the patient's quality of life by reducing symptoms like pain, obstruction, and organ dysfunction.

5.2. Radiation Therapy

Radiation therapy is a critical component of cancer treatment, using high-energy particles or waves to destroy cancer cells. It works by damaging the DNA of cancer cells, inhibiting their ability to replicate and grow.

Radiation can be used in a variety of settings—**curative**, **adjuvant**, or **palliative**—depending on the cancer type, stage, and treatment goals.

5.2.1. Indications for Radiation Therapy

Radiation therapy can be employed in multiple treatment contexts:

Primary Treatment

Radiation therapy is often used as the primary treatment for certain cancers, especially when surgery is not feasible or necessary. It is commonly used in **head and neck cancers**, **prostate cancer**, and certain types of **lymphomas**. In these cases, radiation therapy alone or in combination with chemotherapy can be curative by eliminating the cancer without the need for surgery.

- **Head and Neck Cancers**: For **locally advanced head and neck cancers**, radiation therapy is often combined with chemotherapy to improve locoregional control and survival rates. Studies have demonstrated the efficacy of this combined approach, leading to higher survival rates in cancers such as **nasopharyngeal carcinoma**.

- **Prostate Cancer**: For **early-stage prostate cancer**, radiation is a primary treatment option, especially for patients who are not candidates for surgery. Radiation therapy, particularly in the form of **external beam radiation therapy (EBRT)** or **brachytherapy**, has shown comparable outcomes to surgery in terms of cancer control and long-term survival.

Adjuvant Therapy (Post-Surgery)

Radiation is frequently used as **adjuvant therapy**, meaning it is administered after surgery to destroy any remaining cancer cells and reduce the risk of recurrence. This is common in cancers like **breast cancer** and **rectal cancer**.

- **Breast Cancer**: In **early-stage breast cancer**, radiation therapy is typically delivered after **lumpectomy** (breast-conserving surgery) to reduce local recurrence rates. Multiple studies have shown that radiation therapy following breast-conserving surgery significantly lowers the risk of cancer recurrence and improves survival.
- **Rectal Cancer**: For **locally advanced rectal cancer**, **neoadjuvant radiation therapy** (before surgery) is often used to shrink the tumor, making it easier to remove and increasing the likelihood of sphincter preservation. Postoperative radiation therapy may also be administered to prevent local recurrence.

Palliative Treatment

Radiation is also used **palliatively** to relieve symptoms in advanced cancer cases where a cure is not possible. It can reduce tumor size, alleviate pain from bone metastases, or relieve obstruction caused by tumor growth.

- **Bone Metastases**: In patients with painful bone metastases, a short course of palliative radiation therapy can significantly reduce pain and improve quality of life.
- **Spinal Cord Compression**: Radiation is also crucial in cases of **spinal cord compression** due to metastatic disease, where it can prevent paralysis and provide symptom relief.

5.2.2. Common Side Effects of Radiation Therapy

While radiation therapy is highly effective in targeting cancer cells, it also affects nearby healthy tissues, leading to side effects. The severity of side effects depends on the treatment site, dose, and individual patient factors.

Fatigue

Fatigue is one of the most common side effects of radiation therapy, often developing as treatment progresses and lasting for several weeks or months after treatment ends. Fatigue may result from the body's response to the energy required for repairing damage caused by radiation.

Skin Irritation

Radiation dermatitis is another frequent side effect, especially when the skin is directly exposed to radiation. This can range from mild redness and dryness to more severe peeling or ulceration in cases of high-dose radiation, such as in **breast cancer** or **head and neck cancers**.

Organ-Specific Toxicities

Radiation therapy can cause specific side effects depending on the area of the body being treated:

- **Esophagitis**: In **lung cancer** patients receiving chest radiation, inflammation of the esophagus (**esophagitis**) can occur, leading to pain and difficulty swallowing. This is particularly common when radiation is combined with chemotherapy.
- **Radiation Cystitis**: In patients treated for **prostate cancer** or **pelvic malignancies**, radiation can cause **radiation cystitis**, leading to symptoms such as urinary frequency, urgency, and discomfort.

Long-Term Risks

While radiation therapy is effective in treating cancer, it carries potential long-term risks, including the development of **secondary cancers** and **cardiovascular complications**. For example, **De Ruysscher et al. (2019)** highlighted the increased risk of **secondary lung cancers** and **heart disease** in patients who receive chest irradiation, particularly for **Hodgkin lymphoma** survivors who were treated with high-dose radiation therapy.

5.2.3. Advances in Radiation Therapy Technology

Recent technological advancements have significantly improved the precision and safety of radiation therapy, allowing for higher doses to be delivered to the tumor while minimizing damage to surrounding healthy tissues.

Stereotactic Radiosurgery (SRS)

Stereotactic radiosurgery (SRS) is a highly targeted form of radiation therapy that delivers a single high-dose radiation treatment or a few large fraction doses to a small, localized tumor area. It is most commonly used for:

- **Brain metastases**: SRS allows for precise targeting of brain tumors, minimizing radiation exposure to healthy brain tissue. This technique is highly effective for patients with **brain metastases** from primary cancers such as lung cancer or melanoma, leading to high rates of local tumor control.
- **Early-Stage Lung Cancer**: SRS, also known as **stereotactic body radiation therapy (SBRT)** when applied to areas outside the brain, is increasingly used for **early-stage non-small cell lung cancer (NSCLC)** in patients who are not surgical candidates.

Lagerwaard et al. (2012) demonstrated that **SRS for early-stage lung cancer** resulted in high local control rates, with minimal toxicity and improved overall survival compared to traditional fractionated radiation therapy.

Intensity-Modulated Radiation Therapy (IMRT)

IMRT is an advanced form of radiation therapy that allows for precise dose distribution by modulating the intensity of the radiation beams. It is particularly beneficial in treating tumors located near critical organs, such as:

- **Prostate cancer**: IMRT minimizes radiation exposure to surrounding tissues like the bladder and rectum, reducing the risk of long-term complications such as incontinence and radiation cystitis.
- **Head and neck cancers**: IMRT enables higher radiation doses to be delivered to the tumor while sparing nearby structures such as the salivary glands, reducing the incidence of severe dry mouth (xerostomia).

Proton Beam Therapy

Proton beam therapy is another innovative approach that uses protons instead of traditional X-rays. Protons have a unique physical property known as the **Bragg peak**, which allows them to deposit the majority of their energy directly at the tumor site with minimal exit dose, reducing exposure to healthy tissue.

Pediatric Cancers: Proton therapy is especially valuable in **pediatric cancers**, where reducing radiation exposure to developing tissues is critical for preventing long-term side effects such as growth abnormalities and secondary malignancies.

5.3. Chemotherapy

Chemotherapy is the use of **cytotoxic drugs** designed to kill rapidly dividing cancer cells, a hallmark characteristic of malignancies. While chemotherapy can effectively target and destroy cancer cells, it also affects other rapidly dividing cells in the body, such as those in the bone marrow, gastrointestinal tract, and hair follicles, leading to a wide range of side effects.

Chemotherapy is often used as part of a **multimodal approach** to cancer treatment, alongside surgery and radiation therapy, to improve treatment outcomes. It can be administered as **neoadjuvant therapy** (before surgery) to shrink tumors, **adjuvant therapy** (after surgery) to eliminate residual cancer cells, or as the **primary treatment** for advanced or metastatic cancers.

5.3.1. Common Chemotherapy Drugs and Regimens

The choice of chemotherapy drugs and regimens depends on the type and stage of cancer, as well as the patient's overall health and ability to tolerate treatment. Chemotherapy can be administered as a **single agent** or in **combination regimens** designed to target cancer cells through different mechanisms, thereby increasing the likelihood of treatment success.

Common Chemotherapy Drugs

Chemotherapy drugs are categorized based on their mechanisms of action. The most frequently used classes include:

- **Platinum-Based Agents**: These include **cisplatin** and **carboplatin**, which form cross-links in DNA, preventing cancer cells from replicating. Platinum agents are commonly used in cancers such as **lung, ovarian**, and **testicular cancers**.
- **Taxanes**: **Paclitaxel** and **docetaxel** stabilize microtubules, preventing cell division. They are often used in the treatment of **breast, ovarian, lung**, and **prostate cancers**.
- **Anthracyclines**: Drugs like **doxorubicin** and **epirubicin** interfere with DNA replication by intercalating DNA strands and inhibiting topoisomerase II. Anthracyclines are key drugs in treating **breast cancer, lymphomas**, and **sarcomas**.
- **Antimetabolites**: **5-fluorouracil (5-FU)** and **methotrexate** disrupt DNA synthesis by mimicking normal cellular metabolites. These agents are commonly used in the treatment of **colorectal, breast**, and **gastric cancers**.

Common Chemotherapy Regimens

Chemotherapy regimens are often designed to combine drugs with complementary mechanisms of action, enhancing the likelihood of eradicating cancer cells. Some widely used regimens include:

- **FOLFOX (folinic acid, fluorouracil, oxaliplatin)**: Used in the treatment of **colorectal cancer**, this regimen combines an antimetabolite (fluorouracil), a platinum-based agent (oxaliplatin), and folinic acid to enhance the effect of fluorouracil. Studies have demonstrated that FOLFOX improves survival rates in patients with stage III and IV colorectal cancer, both in the adjuvant and palliative settings.
- **CHOP (cyclophosphamide, doxorubicin, vincristine, prednisone)**: A standard regimen for **non-Hodgkin lymphoma**, CHOP combines four drugs that work synergistically to target rapidly dividing cells. **Cyclophosphamide** and **doxorubicin** damage DNA, **vincristine** disrupts microtubule formation, and **prednisone** is a corticosteroid that helps reduce inflammation and enhance chemotherapy efficacy.
- **AC-T (doxorubicin, cyclophosphamide, paclitaxel)**: Commonly used in **breast cancer**, this regimen is delivered in sequential phases, with the anthracycline (doxorubicin) and cyclophosphamide given first, followed by the taxane (paclitaxel) to maximize therapeutic benefit.

5.3.2. Monitoring for Chemotherapy Toxicity

Chemotherapy, while effective, is associated with **significant toxicity** because it also affects healthy cells that divide rapidly. To minimize these toxic effects, patients undergoing chemotherapy require regular monitoring of their health, especially blood counts and organ function. Common toxicities include:

Myelosuppression

- **Myelosuppression**, or suppression of bone marrow activity, is one of the most common side effects of chemotherapy. This can lead to **neutropenia** (low white blood cell counts), **anemia** (low red blood cell counts), and **thrombocytopenia** (low platelet counts). Patients with neutropenia are at an increased risk of **infections**.
    - **Febrile neutropenia**, a potentially life-threatening complication, occurs when a patient with neutropenia develops a fever, indicating an infection. It requires immediate medical intervention. In high-risk patients, **granulocyte colony-stimulating factors (G-CSF)**, such as **filgrastim**, can be administered to stimulate white blood cell production and reduce the risk of neutropenia.

Nausea and Vomiting

- Chemotherapy-induced **nausea and vomiting (CINV)** are common and can significantly impact a patient's quality of life. Antiemetic medications such as **ondansetron**, **aprepitant**, and **dexamethasone** are commonly used to prevent or manage nausea and vomiting during chemotherapy.

Neuropathy

- **Peripheral neuropathy** is a common side effect of drugs like **taxanes** and **platinum-based agents**. Patients may experience numbness, tingling, or pain in the hands and feet, which can become debilitating over time. **Dose adjustments** or changes in treatment may be necessary if neuropathy becomes severe.

Organ Toxicities

- Chemotherapy can cause damage to organs such as the **heart**, **kidneys**, and **liver**. **Anthracyclines**, such as doxorubicin, are associated with **cardiotoxicity**, which can lead to heart failure if cumulative doses are too high. Regular monitoring of **cardiac function** using **echocardiograms** or **MUGA scans** is essential in patients receiving anthracyclines.
- **Nephrotoxicity** is a concern with drugs like **cisplatin**, which can impair kidney function. Patients undergoing chemotherapy with nephrotoxic drugs need regular monitoring of **renal function** through serum creatinine and electrolyte levels to detect early signs of kidney damage.

Long-Term Effects

- In addition to acute side effects, chemotherapy can cause long-term complications, such as **secondary malignancies**. Some chemotherapy agents, such as **alkylating agents**, increase the risk of developing secondary cancers like **leukemia**. Patients require long-term follow-up to monitor for these potential late effects.

5.3. Immunotherapy

Immunotherapy has emerged as a groundbreaking approach in cancer treatment, fundamentally altering the landscape for cancers that have been historically difficult to treat with conventional therapies like chemotherapy and radiation.

By leveraging the body's immune system to recognize and destroy cancer cells, immunotherapy offers a highly targeted treatment strategy that can produce durable responses. Two of the most impactful immunotherapy modalities in recent years are **checkpoint inhibitors** and **chimeric antigen receptor T-cell (CAR-T) therapy**.

5.3.1. Checkpoint Inhibitors

Checkpoint inhibitors represent a class of immunotherapy drugs that have revolutionized the treatment of several cancers, including **non-small cell lung cancer (NSCLC)**, **melanoma**, **renal cell carcinoma**, and more. These drugs target immune checkpoints—proteins that regulate immune responses—to prevent cancer cells from evading detection by the immune system.

Mechanism of Action

Cancer cells exploit immune checkpoint pathways, such as **PD-1/PD-L1** and **CTLA-4**, to avoid immune surveillance. Normally, these pathways act as brakes on the immune system to prevent it from attacking normal cells. However, many cancers overexpress **PD-L1** or other checkpoint proteins, effectively turning off T cells and allowing cancer cells to proliferate unchecked.

Checkpoint inhibitors like **pembrolizumab (Keytruda)** and **nivolumab (Opdivo)** work by blocking these checkpoint pathways, thus restoring T cell activity and enabling the immune system to recognize and destroy cancer cells.

Proven Efficacy in Cancer Treatment

- **Non-Small Cell Lung Cancer (NSCLC)**: Checkpoint inhibitors have significantly improved outcomes in patients with NSCLC, particularly those who express high levels of **PD-L1**. In a landmark study by **Reck et al. (2016)**, pembrolizumab was compared to standard chemotherapy in patients with **PD-L1-positive NSCLC**. The study found that pembrolizumab significantly improved **overall survival (OS)** and **progression-free survival (PFS)** compared to chemotherapy, particularly in patients whose tumors had high PD-L1 expression. This trial established pembrolizumab as a frontline treatment option for patients with PD-L1-positive advanced NSCLC.
- **Melanoma**: Checkpoint inhibitors have also transformed the treatment of **melanoma**, especially in advanced stages where conventional therapies had limited efficacy. Drugs like nivolumab and pembrolizumab have demonstrated durable responses and

prolonged survival in metastatic melanoma. Studies have shown that these therapies significantly improve **five-year survival rates**, a remarkable achievement in a historically difficult-to-treat cancer.
- **Renal Cell Carcinoma (RCC)**: For patients with **advanced renal cell carcinoma**, checkpoint inhibitors, either alone or in combination with other therapies (such as targeted therapies), have shown superior outcomes compared to older treatments. For instance, the combination of nivolumab and **ipilimumab (Yervoy)**, a CTLA-4 inhibitor, has demonstrated a significant survival benefit in metastatic RCC patients, particularly those with intermediate- or poor-risk disease.

Toxicities and Management

While checkpoint inhibitors have produced impressive results, they are associated with **immune-related adverse events (irAEs)** due to the activation of the immune system. These toxicities can affect various organs and include:

- **Colitis**: Inflammation of the colon can lead to severe diarrhea and abdominal pain.
- **Hepatitis**: Liver inflammation can cause elevated liver enzymes and jaundice.
- **Pneumonitis**: Inflammation of lung tissue can cause shortness of breath and cough.
- **Endocrinopathies**: Hypothyroidism, adrenal insufficiency, and diabetes can occur due to immune-mediated damage to endocrine organs.

Managing these toxicities often requires immunosuppressive treatment with **corticosteroids** or other immunomodulatory agents. Early recognition and intervention are key to minimizing long-term damage from irAEs.

5.3.2. CAR-T Cell Therapy

Chimeric Antigen Receptor T-cell (CAR-T) therapy is a novel form of immunotherapy that has shown remarkable efficacy in certain hematologic cancers, particularly in patients with **relapsed or refractory disease** who have exhausted other treatment options. CAR-T therapy involves engineering a patient's own T cells to specifically recognize and attack cancer cells.

Mechanism of Action

In CAR-T therapy, a patient's T cells are collected and genetically modified in a laboratory to express a **chimeric antigen receptor (CAR)**, which enables the T cells to target a specific antigen present on cancer cells. These modified T cells are then expanded and reinfused into the patient, where they can recognize and destroy cancer cells expressing the target antigen.

One of the most successful targets for CAR-T therapy has been **CD19**, a protein commonly found on **B-cell malignancies** such as **acute lymphoblastic leukemia (ALL)** and **diffuse large B-cell lymphoma (DLBCL)**.

Proven Efficacy in Hematologic Malignancies

- **Acute Lymphoblastic Leukemia (ALL)**: CAR-T therapy has shown exceptional results in patients with **relapsed or refractory ALL**, particularly in pediatric and young adult populations. **Maude et al. (2018)** demonstrated the efficacy of **tisagenlecleucel**, a CAR-T therapy targeting CD19, in achieving high remission rates in children and young adults with relapsed ALL. In their study, **tisagenlecleucel** induced complete remission in up to 81% of patients, a remarkable outcome for a population with otherwise poor prognosis.
- **Diffuse Large B-Cell Lymphoma (DLBCL)**: CAR-T therapies have also been approved for the treatment of **refractory DLBCL**. Patients who had failed previous lines of chemotherapy showed significant response rates after receiving CAR-T therapy, with many achieving durable remissions.

Limitations and Toxicities

Despite its groundbreaking efficacy, CAR-T therapy is associated with significant toxicities that limit its use to specialized centers capable of managing severe side effects:

- **Cytokine Release Syndrome (CRS)**: One of the most common and serious side effects of CAR-T therapy is **cytokine release syndrome (CRS)**, a systemic inflammatory response caused by the rapid activation and proliferation of T cells. CRS can manifest with fever, hypotension, and multi-organ dysfunction, and in severe cases, it can be life-threatening. **Tocilizumab**, an IL-6 receptor antagonist, is commonly used to manage CRS, alongside corticosteroids in more severe cases.
- **Neurotoxicity**: Another significant toxicity is **immune effector cell-associated neurotoxicity syndrome (ICANS)**, which can present with confusion, seizures, or even coma. Neurotoxicity often requires prompt intervention with steroids and supportive care to prevent long-term sequelae.
- **Access and Cost**: CAR-T therapy is highly complex and expensive, requiring sophisticated laboratory facilities and extended hospital stays for monitoring. As a result, it is currently only available in specialized centers with experience in managing its toxicities.

5.4. Targeted Therapy

Targeted therapies are a class of cancer treatments specifically designed to interfere with molecular pathways critical for the growth and survival of cancer cells. Unlike chemotherapy, which indiscriminately targets all rapidly dividing cells, including healthy ones, targeted therapy is directed at specific proteins, genes, or other molecules that are unique to cancer cells.

5.4.1. Mechanism of Action: Targeting Cancer-Specific Molecules

Targeted therapies work by blocking specific molecules or pathways that cancer cells depend on for growth, proliferation, and survival. These targets may include mutant proteins, overexpressed receptors, or other dysregulated cellular processes specific to cancer cells. By interrupting these critical pathways, targeted therapies can halt tumor progression or induce cancer cell death.

5.4. 2. Types of Targeted Therapies

Tyrosine kinase inhibitors (TKIs) are small molecules that block the activity of tyrosine kinases, enzymes that play a crucial role in signaling pathways controlling cell division, growth, and survival. Mutations or abnormal activation of these kinases can drive cancer progression, making them ideal therapeutic targets.

- **Imatinib (Gleevec)**: One of the first and most successful TKIs, **imatinib** revolutionized the treatment of **chronic myeloid leukemia (CML)** by targeting the **BCR-ABL fusion protein**, an abnormal tyrosine kinase produced by the Philadelphia chromosome in CML cells. Imatinib's development marked a significant milestone in precision oncology, converting a once-fatal disease into a manageable chronic condition for many patients. Clinical studies have shown that long-term treatment with imatinib leads to durable remissions and significantly improved survival in CML patients.
- **EGFR Inhibitors (Erlotinib and Gefitinib)**: In **non-small cell lung cancer (NSCLC)**, mutations in the **epidermal growth factor receptor (EGFR)** gene drive tumor growth by continuously activating the EGFR signaling pathway. **Erlotinib** and **gefitinib** are TKIs that inhibit EGFR, effectively blocking the pathway and inducing tumor shrinkage in patients with **EGFR-mutated NSCLC**. Studies have shown that patients with these mutations experience significantly improved **progression-free survival (PFS)** compared to those treated with traditional chemotherapy.
- **ALK Inhibitors (Crizotinib)**: Another major advancement in lung cancer treatment is the development of **ALK inhibitors** like **crizotinib**, which targets tumors with rearrangements in the **anaplastic lymphoma kinase (ALK)** gene. In the pivotal study by **Solomon et al. (2014)**, crizotinib demonstrated superior progression-free survival compared to chemotherapy in patients with **ALK-positive NSCLC**, establishing it as a first-line therapy in this population.

Monoclonal antibodies are laboratory-made molecules that can bind to specific antigens on the surface of cancer cells, blocking critical signaling pathways, inducing immune responses, or delivering cytotoxic agents directly to cancer cells. These therapies have been particularly effective in cancers that overexpress specific proteins or receptors.

- **Trastuzumab (Herceptin)**: **Trastuzumab** targets the **HER2** protein, which is overexpressed in approximately 20% of **breast cancers** and some gastric cancers. HER2-positive breast cancers tend to be more aggressive, but trastuzumab has dramatically improved outcomes in these patients. By binding to HER2, trastuzumab blocks the receptor's signaling and recruits immune cells to attack the tumor. Long-term studies have shown that adding trastuzumab to chemotherapy improves both **overall survival (OS)** and **disease-free survival (DFS)** in HER2-positive breast cancer patients.
- **Rituximab (Rituxan)**: In **B-cell lymphomas**, **rituximab** targets the **CD20** protein found on the surface of B cells. By binding to CD20, rituximab induces immune-mediated destruction of cancerous B cells. When added to chemotherapy regimens like **CHOP**,

rituximab has significantly improved survival rates in patients with **non-Hodgkin lymphoma**, particularly **diffuse large B-cell lymphoma (DLBCL)**.

5.4.3. Specific Targeted Treatments

The advent of **precision medicine** has enabled clinicians to select therapies based on the specific genetic and molecular characteristics of a patient's tumor. By identifying key mutations or biomarkers, oncologists can tailor treatment to maximize efficacy and minimize unnecessary toxicity.

BRAF Inhibitors in Melanoma

- In **melanoma**, approximately 50% of patients harbor mutations in the **BRAF** gene, specifically the **BRAF V600E mutation**, which drives uncontrolled cell growth through the MAPK signaling pathway. **BRAF inhibitors**, such as **vemurafenib** and **dabrafenib**, target the mutated BRAF protein, blocking this pathway and leading to tumor regression. Studies have shown that BRAF inhibitors, especially when combined with **MEK inhibitors**, significantly improve progression-free survival and overall survival in patients with **BRAF-mutated melanoma**.

PARP Inhibitors in BRCA-Mutated Cancers

- **Poly (ADP-ribose) polymerase (PARP) inhibitors** have emerged as a powerful tool in cancers with **BRCA1/2 mutations**, which impair DNA repair mechanisms in cells. PARP inhibitors, such as **olaparib** and **rucaparib**, further inhibit DNA repair, leading to the accumulation of DNA damage in cancer cells and eventually cell death. These drugs have been particularly effective in **BRCA-mutated ovarian and breast cancers**. In a clinical trial conducted by **Robson et al. (2017)**, **olaparib** significantly prolonged **progression-free survival** in patients with **BRCA-mutated breast cancer**, establishing it as an essential therapy in this population.

5.4.4. Challenges and Future Directions in Targeted Therapy

While targeted therapies have revolutionized cancer treatment, they are not without challenges:

- **Resistance**: One of the primary challenges with targeted therapies is the development of **drug resistance**. Cancer cells can evolve and find alternative pathways to survive, diminishing the long-term efficacy of targeted drugs. For example, in patients treated with EGFR inhibitors, secondary mutations (e.g., **T790M mutation**) often emerge, leading to resistance. Newer generations of TKIs, such as **osimertinib**, have been developed to overcome these resistance mechanisms.
- **Toxicity**: Although targeted therapies are generally less toxic than chemotherapy, they are not without side effects. **Cardiotoxicity** with trastuzumab and **dermatologic toxicities** with EGFR inhibitors are well-documented adverse effects that require monitoring and management.

- **Cost and Accessibility**: Targeted therapies can be costly, and their accessibility may be limited in certain healthcare systems or geographic regions. Ensuring equitable access to these life-saving therapies remains a critical challenge in oncology.

5.5. Hormonal Therapy

Hormonal therapy is a critical treatment modality for cancers that rely on hormones for growth and survival. This approach is primarily used in **breast cancer** and **prostate cancer**, where hormone receptors drive the proliferation of cancer cells. By blocking or reducing hormone levels, hormonal therapies aim to inhibit tumor growth and prevent recurrence, offering a less toxic alternative to chemotherapy for certain patients.

5.5.1. Hormonal Therapy for Breast Cancer

Breast cancer is often driven by estrogen, particularly in **estrogen receptor-positive (ER+)** tumors, which account for approximately 70% of all breast cancers. In ER+ breast cancer, estrogen binds to the estrogen receptors on cancer cells, promoting cell division and tumor growth. **Hormonal therapy** in these patients is aimed at blocking estrogen signaling, thereby slowing or stopping cancer progression.

Estrogen Receptor Modulators

One of the mainstays of hormonal therapy in ER+ breast cancer is the use of **selective estrogen receptor modulators (SERMs)** like **tamoxifen**. Tamoxifen works by competitively binding to estrogen receptors, blocking estrogen's ability to activate these receptors in breast tissue. As a result, tamoxifen reduces the growth-stimulating effects of estrogen on cancer cells.

- **Tamoxifen's Proven Efficacy**: Tamoxifen has been extensively studied in both early and advanced-stage breast cancer. According to the **Early Breast Cancer Trialists' Collaborative Group (2011)**, five years of tamoxifen therapy reduces the risk of **breast cancer recurrence** by approximately 50% in hormone receptor-positive patients. Additionally, tamoxifen reduces the risk of **breast cancer mortality** by approximately 30%, making it one of the most effective adjuvant therapies for ER+ breast cancer.
- **Long-Term Benefits**: The benefits of tamoxifen extend well beyond the initial five years of therapy. Studies have shown that patients who complete five years of tamoxifen continue to experience a reduced risk of recurrence and death from breast cancer for many years after stopping the medication.

Aromatase Inhibitors

In postmenopausal women, **aromatase inhibitors** (AIs) such as **anastrozole**, **letrozole**, and **exemestane** are frequently used in place of tamoxifen. Aromatase inhibitors work by blocking the enzyme **aromatase**, which converts androgens to estrogens in peripheral tissues. By reducing estrogen levels in postmenopausal women, AIs significantly decrease the availability of estrogen to stimulate cancer growth.

- **Superiority in Postmenopausal Women**: Studies have demonstrated that aromatase inhibitors are more effective than tamoxifen in preventing recurrence in postmenopausal women with ER+ breast cancer. They are typically used as adjuvant therapy for 5-10 years, either alone or in sequence with tamoxifen. A meta-analysis of several clinical trials revealed that patients on AIs had a lower risk of recurrence compared to those on tamoxifen, particularly in the first few years of treatment.

Side Effects of Hormonal Therapy in Breast Cancer

While hormonal therapies like tamoxifen and AIs are effective, they are associated with specific side effects:

- **Tamoxifen**: Common side effects include **hot flashes, vaginal dryness**, and an increased risk of **venous thromboembolism** and **endometrial cancer** due to its partial agonist effect on the endometrium.
- **Aromatase Inhibitors**: AIs are associated with **bone density loss**, leading to an increased risk of osteoporosis and fractures. Patients on AIs are often monitored for bone health, and calcium/vitamin D supplementation or bisphosphonates may be recommended to mitigate bone loss.

5.5.2. Hormonal Therapy for Prostate Cancer

Prostate cancer is highly dependent on **androgens** (male hormones such as testosterone) for growth. **Androgen deprivation therapy (ADT)** is the cornerstone of treatment for **metastatic** and advanced prostate cancer. ADT works by reducing the production of androgens or blocking their effects on prostate cancer cells, thereby slowing the progression of the disease.

Mechanism of Androgen Deprivation Therapy (ADT)

There are several approaches to androgen deprivation therapy:

- **Luteinizing Hormone-Releasing Hormone (LHRH) Agonists and Antagonists**: These drugs, such as **leuprolide** and **degarelix**, reduce testosterone production by suppressing signals from the pituitary gland that stimulate the testes to produce testosterone.
- **Anti-Androgens**: Drugs like **bicalutamide** and **enzalutamide** block androgen receptors on prostate cancer cells, preventing testosterone from binding and activating the receptor. This directly inhibits the cancer-promoting effects of androgens.

Combining ADT with Other Therapies

ADT is often used in combination with other treatments, such as radiation or newer anti-androgen drugs, for improved outcomes. One of the most significant advancements in prostate cancer therapy has been the combination of ADT with **abiraterone**, a drug that blocks **androgen synthesis** not only in the testes but also in the adrenal glands and prostate tumor cells.

- **Abiraterone in Castration-Sensitive Prostate Cancer**: Crawford et al. (2019) demonstrated that adding **abiraterone** to ADT significantly improves **overall survival** and **progression-free survival** in men with **metastatic castration-sensitive prostate cancer**. This combination therapy has become a standard of care for patients with advanced disease, significantly delaying disease progression and extending survival.

Androgen Deprivation Therapy in Different Prostate Cancer Stages

- **Localized Prostate Cancer**: In patients with **intermediate- or high-risk localized prostate cancer**, ADT is sometimes used in combination with **radiation therapy** to enhance the effectiveness of the treatment.
- **Metastatic Prostate Cancer**: For patients with **metastatic prostate cancer**, ADT remains the primary therapy. Over time, however, prostate cancer can become resistant to ADT, a condition known as **castration-resistant prostate cancer (CRPC)**. In these cases, second-line hormonal therapies, such as **enzalutamide** and **abiraterone**, are used to further inhibit androgen signaling and prolong survival.

Side Effects of ADT

Androgen deprivation therapy, while effective in controlling prostate cancer, can cause significant side effects due to the reduction of testosterone levels:

- **Hot Flashes**: A common and often bothersome side effect for men undergoing ADT.
- **Decreased Libido and Erectile Dysfunction**: Lowered testosterone can lead to sexual dysfunction, which may significantly impact quality of life.
- **Bone Density Loss**: Similar to aromatase inhibitors in breast cancer, ADT is associated with bone loss, increasing the risk of fractures.
- **Metabolic Effects**: ADT can contribute to weight gain, loss of muscle mass, insulin resistance, and an increased risk of **cardiovascular disease**.

5.6. Precision Medicine in Cancer Care

Precision medicine has transformed cancer treatment by tailoring therapies based on the **genetic and molecular characteristics** of an individual's tumor, rather than relying solely on the tumor's anatomical location or histology.

5.6.1. An Overview of Precision Medicine

Traditional cancer treatments, such as chemotherapy and radiation, are generally based on the tumor's location and histological appearance. While these treatments can be effective, they often have non-specific effects, leading to significant toxicity by damaging both cancerous and normal cells. In contrast, precision medicine targets the molecular abnormalities specific to cancer cells, leading to **more personalized and precise treatment plans**.

By using molecular profiling techniques like **next-generation sequencing (NGS)**, oncologists can analyze the genetic makeup of a tumor, identifying mutations, gene amplifications, or protein overexpression that are driving cancer progression. This information can then be used to select **targeted therapies** or **immunotherapies** that specifically attack the cancer's vulnerabilities, sparing healthy tissue and reducing overall treatment toxicity.

5.6.2. Molecular Profiling and Personalized Treatment Plans

Molecular profiling is now routinely integrated into the treatment planning for several cancers, including **non-small cell lung cancer (NSCLC), colorectal cancer, melanoma, breast cancer**, and **prostate cancer**. By identifying genetic mutations or alterations in these cancers, oncologists can prescribe therapies that are specifically designed to target those molecular drivers. This approach has revolutionized cancer care, leading to better outcomes and more durable responses compared to traditional chemotherapy.

NSCLC: EGFR, ALK, and PD-L1 Mutations

Non-small cell lung cancer (NSCLC) has become a model for the application of precision medicine. Molecular profiling is now a standard part of the diagnostic process for NSCLC, enabling clinicians to identify mutations in genes such as **EGFR (epidermal growth factor receptor), ALK (anaplastic lymphoma kinase), ROS1**, and **BRAF**. These mutations are targeted by **tyrosine kinase inhibitors (TKIs)**, which block the aberrant signaling pathways that drive cancer growth.

- **EGFR Mutations**: Patients with **EGFR-mutated NSCLC** are treated with **EGFR inhibitors** like **erlotinib, gefitinib**, or **osimertinib**, which have shown superior outcomes compared to traditional chemotherapy. In a study by **Paz-Ares et al. (2018)**, NSCLC patients with **EGFR mutations** had significantly improved **progression-free survival (PFS)** and **overall survival (OS)** when treated with EGFR inhibitors.
- **ALK and ROS1 Rearrangements**: Similarly, patients with **ALK** or **ROS1** gene rearrangements are treated with **ALK inhibitors** such as **crizotinib** or **alectinib**. These targeted therapies have led to marked improvements in outcomes, with fewer side effects compared to chemotherapy.
- **PD-L1 Expression**: Immunotherapy has also played a pivotal role in precision medicine for NSCLC. **PD-L1 expression**, which allows cancer cells to evade immune detection, can be targeted by **checkpoint inhibitors** such as **pembrolizumab** and **nivolumab**. Patients with high PD-L1 expression benefit significantly from these therapies, with prolonged survival compared to traditional treatments.

Colorectal Cancer: KRAS and BRAF Mutations

Colorectal cancer treatment has also been transformed by molecular profiling. The identification of **KRAS, NRAS**, and **BRAF** mutations in colorectal tumors has allowed for more precise treatment plans.

- **KRAS/NRAS Mutations**: Patients with **KRAS** or **NRAS** mutations do not respond to **anti-EGFR therapies** (such as cetuximab and panitumumab), and therefore, these therapies are avoided in patients with these mutations. Precision medicine ensures that only patients likely to benefit from targeted therapies receive them, preventing unnecessary toxicity in patients unlikely to respond.
- **BRAF Mutations**: For patients with **BRAF-mutated colorectal cancer**, particularly those with the **BRAF V600E mutation**, targeted therapies such as **BRAF inhibitors** (e.g., vemurafenib) in combination with other agents like **MEK inhibitors** have shown promising results. Studies have demonstrated improved **response rates** and **survival** when these targeted therapies are used in patients with specific molecular profiles.

Melanoma: BRAF Mutations

In **melanoma**, precision medicine has been particularly successful in treating patients with **BRAF mutations**, which are present in about 50% of advanced melanoma cases.

- **BRAF Inhibitors**: **Vemurafenib** and **dabrafenib** are BRAF inhibitors that target the **BRAF V600E mutation**, which drives melanoma progression by continuously activating the MAPK signaling pathway. These therapies have been shown to shrink tumors and improve survival, particularly when combined with **MEK inhibitors**, which block a downstream component of the same pathway, further enhancing the efficacy of the treatment.
- **Durable Responses**: Studies have shown that patients with BRAF-mutated melanoma treated with **BRAF inhibitors** experience high **response rates** and durable tumor control. However, the combination of BRAF and MEK inhibitors has been found to further reduce the risk of drug resistance, which can occur with monotherapy.

5.6.3. Advantages of Precision Medicine in Cancer Care

Increased Efficacy and Survival

Precision medicine allows for more effective treatments, as therapies are tailored to the specific molecular drivers of a patient's cancer. By targeting these specific mutations, patients often experience **improved outcomes**, including **higher response rates**, **longer progression-free survival**, and **better overall survival**. This has been especially evident in cancers like **NSCLC**, **melanoma**, and **colorectal cancer**, where targeted therapies have replaced or augmented traditional chemotherapy.

Reduced Toxicity

Because precision medicine focuses on the molecular drivers of cancer, it often spares normal cells, reducing the **collateral damage** that is common with chemotherapy and radiation. Patients treated with targeted therapies or immunotherapies tend to experience fewer severe side effects, making treatment more tolerable and improving quality of life during treatment.

Prevention of Overtreatment

Molecular profiling ensures that patients are only treated with therapies they are likely to benefit from. This prevents overtreatment and avoids exposing patients to ineffective treatments, which may carry unnecessary toxicity. For example, **anti-EGFR therapies** are only used in colorectal cancer patients without **KRAS** or **NRAS mutations**, ensuring that resources are directed toward those most likely to benefit.

5.6.4. Challenges in Precision Medicine

While precision medicine offers significant advantages, it also faces challenges:

- **Cost and Accessibility**: Comprehensive tumor profiling and targeted therapies can be expensive, limiting their availability in some healthcare systems or geographic regions. Ensuring access to these life-saving treatments is a major challenge in global cancer care.
- **Resistance Mechanisms**: While targeted therapies are highly effective initially, many cancers develop **resistance** over time by finding alternative pathways to grow and survive. Research is ongoing to overcome resistance and extend the efficacy of targeted therapies.
- **Tumor Heterogeneity**: Cancers are often heterogeneous, meaning different areas of the tumor may harbor different mutations. This can complicate treatment, as a therapy targeting one mutation may not be effective against all the tumor cells.

5.7. Latest Advances in Cancer Treatment

Significant strides in cancer treatment have emerged in recent years, with new therapies pushing the boundaries of how cancer is managed. Among the most exciting innovations are **antibody-drug conjugates (ADCs)** and **mRNA vaccines**, both of which represent cutting-edge approaches to targeting cancer cells while minimizing harm to normal tissues.

5.7.1. Antibody-Drug Conjugates (ADCs)

Antibody-drug conjugates (ADCs) are a promising class of targeted cancer therapies that combine the specificity of **monoclonal antibodies** with the cytotoxic power of **chemotherapy drugs**. These drugs consist of three main components: a monoclonal antibody that binds specifically to antigens expressed on the surface of cancer cells, a cytotoxic drug (chemotherapy), and a linker that connects the two. This structure allows ADCs to selectively deliver chemotherapy directly to cancer cells, sparing healthy tissues and reducing the systemic toxicity typically associated with traditional chemotherapy.

Mechanism of Action

ADCs work by targeting specific antigens on cancer cells. Once the monoclonal antibody component binds to its antigen on the cancer cell, the entire ADC is internalized into the cell. Once inside, the linker is cleaved, releasing the cytotoxic drug directly into the cancer cell, leading to its destruction. This targeted delivery limits the exposure of healthy cells to chemotherapy, thereby reducing the risk of side effects.

Trastuzumab Emtansine (T-DM1)

One of the most successful examples of an ADC is **trastuzumab emtansine (T-DM1)**, which is used to treat **HER2-positive breast cancer**. HER2 is a protein that promotes the growth of cancer cells and is overexpressed in about 20% of breast cancers. **Trastuzumab**, a monoclonal antibody targeting HER2, is linked to **emtansine**, a potent chemotherapy drug. This combination allows trastuzumab to deliver emtansine directly to HER2-positive cancer cells.

- **Clinical Efficacy**: In a pivotal study by **Verma et al. (2012)**, T-DM1 was shown to significantly improve **progression-free survival (PFS)** and overall survival compared to traditional chemotherapy in patients with **HER2-positive metastatic breast cancer**. The study demonstrated that T-DM1 led to a median PFS of 9.6 months, compared to 6.4 months with conventional chemotherapy. These results solidified T-DM1 as a critical therapy for HER2-positive breast cancer, particularly for patients whose disease has progressed after prior HER2-targeted therapies.
- **Reduced Toxicity**: Importantly, the side effect profile of T-DM1 is more favorable than traditional chemotherapy, with fewer cases of severe nausea, vomiting, and hair loss. This improvement in quality of life is a significant advantage for patients undergoing long-term treatment.

Expansion of ADCs to Other Cancers

Beyond HER2-positive breast cancer, ADCs are being developed and tested in other cancer types, including **lung cancer**, **lymphomas**, and **bladder cancer**. For example, **enfortumab vedotin**, an ADC targeting **Nectin-4** (a protein highly expressed in **urothelial carcinoma**), has shown promising results in **advanced bladder cancer**. Similarly, **brentuximab vedotin**, an ADC targeting **CD30**, has been used effectively in **Hodgkin lymphoma** and **anaplastic large cell lymphoma**

5.7.2. mRNA Vaccines and Their Potential Role in Oncology

The success of **mRNA vaccines** during the COVID-19 pandemic has sparked tremendous interest in applying this technology to cancer treatment. **mRNA vaccines** work by encoding antigens—proteins that stimulate an immune response—into a strand of messenger RNA (mRNA). Once administered, the mRNA is taken up by cells, which then produce the encoded antigen and present it to the immune system, triggering a targeted immune response against cells expressing that antigen. In oncology, mRNA vaccines are designed to encode **tumor-specific antigens**, encouraging the immune system to recognize and attack cancer cells.

Mechanism of Action

In cancer, the immune system often fails to recognize tumor cells as threats, allowing cancer to grow unchecked. mRNA vaccines offer a way to reprogram the immune system to detect and destroy cancer cells by presenting **neoantigens**, which are abnormal proteins generated by cancer cells due to mutations. These neoantigens are unique to cancer cells and can be used to "train" the immune system to distinguish between healthy and malignant cells.

Personalized mRNA Vaccines

One of the most promising applications of mRNA technology in cancer treatment is the development of **personalized mRNA vaccines**. By sequencing a patient's tumor, scientists can identify neoantigens specific to that individual's cancer and design a custom mRNA vaccine that encodes those neoantigens. The vaccine is then used to stimulate a patient-specific immune response, targeting the cancer cells more precisely.

- **Clinical Trials in Melanoma**: Early studies have shown encouraging results. For instance, in a study by **Sahin et al. (2020)**, **personalized mRNA vaccines** were tested in patients with advanced **melanoma**. The vaccines were designed to target neoantigens unique to each patient's tumor. Results indicated that some patients experienced **durable responses** to the vaccine, with their immune systems launching targeted attacks against the cancer cells. While still in its early stages, this approach shows significant promise for the future of personalized cancer immunotherapy.

Advantages of mRNA Vaccines

- **Rapid Development**: One of the key advantages of mRNA vaccines is the speed with which they can be designed and produced. Because they are synthesized in a laboratory without the need for biological materials, mRNA vaccines can be rapidly developed and tailored to individual patients.
- **Flexibility**: The mRNA platform is highly flexible, meaning it can be adapted to target a wide range of cancer types by encoding different tumor antigens. This versatility makes mRNA vaccines an attractive option for both personalized and universal cancer immunotherapies.
- **Immune Potency**: mRNA vaccines have been shown to generate strong immune responses, particularly when combined with other immunotherapy agents such as **checkpoint inhibitors**. By stimulating both **T cells** and **antibody responses**, mRNA vaccines can offer a comprehensive attack on cancer cells.

Challenges and Future Directions

While mRNA vaccines hold tremendous potential, several challenges remain:

- **Tumor Heterogeneity**: One of the major challenges is **tumor heterogeneity**, where different regions of the same tumor may have different mutations. This makes it difficult to design a single vaccine that can target all cancer cells effectively.
- **Immune Evasion**: Some tumors have developed mechanisms to evade the immune system, making it more difficult for vaccines to generate an effective response. Research is ongoing to combine mRNA vaccines with other immunotherapies, such as **PD-1/PD-L1 inhibitors**, to overcome this issue.

References

- Siegel RL, Miller KD, Jemal A. Cancer statistics, 2022. *CA Cancer J Clin.* 2022;72(1):7-33.
- De Ruysscher D, Niedermann G, Burnet NG, et al. Radiotherapy toxicity. *Nat Rev Dis Primers.* 2019;5(1):13.
- Lagerwaard FJ, Haasbeek CJ, Smit EF, Slotman BJ, Senan S. Outcomes of stereotactic radiotherapy for centrally located early-stage lung cancer. *J Thorac Oncol.* 2012;7(10):1507-1513.
- Cohen L, de Moor CA, Eisenberg P, et al. Chemotherapy-induced nausea and vomiting: incidence and impact on patient quality of life at community oncology settings. *Support Care Cancer.* 2017;25(7):2159-2166.
- Reck M, Rodríguez-Abreu D, Robinson AG, et al. Pembrolizumab versus chemotherapy for PD-L1–positive non–small-cell lung cancer. *N Engl J Med.* 2016;375(19):1823-1833.
- Maude SL, Laetsch TW, Buechner J, et al. Tisagenlecleucel in children and young adults with B-cell lymphoblastic leukemia. *N Engl J Med.* 2018;378(5):439-448.
- Solomon BJ, Mok T, Kim DW, et al. First-line crizotinib versus chemotherapy in ALK-positive lung cancer. *N Engl J Med.* 2014;371(23):2167-2177.
- Robson M, Im SA, Senkus E, et al. Olaparib for metastatic breast cancer in patients with a germline BRCA mutation. *N Engl J Med.* 2017;377(6):523-533.
- Early Breast Cancer Trialists' Collaborative Group (EBCTCG). Effects of chemotherapy and hormonal therapy for early breast cancer on recurrence and 15-year survival: an overview of the randomized trials. *Lancet.* 2011;365(9472):1687-1717.
- Crawford ED, Petrylak DP, Shore N, et al. Androgen-targeted therapies in men with prostate cancer: evolving practice and future considerations. *Prostate Cancer Prostatic Dis.* 2019;22(1):24-38.
- Paz-Ares L, Tan EH, O'Byrne K, et al. First-line nivolumab plus ipilimumab in metastatic non-small-cell lung cancer. *N Engl J Med.* 2018;379(14):1380-1391.
- Verma S, Miles D, Gianni L, et al. Trastuzumab emtansine for HER2-positive advanced breast cancer. *N Engl J Med.* 2012;367(19):1783-1791.
- Sahin U, Derhovanessian E, Miller M, et al. Personalized RNA mutanome vaccines mobilize poly-specific therapeutic immunity against cancer. *Nature.* 2020;547(7662):222-226.

Part II: NCCN Cancer Treatment Guidelines

Chapter 6: NCCN Treatment Guidelines for Common Cancers

The **National Comprehensive Cancer Network (NCCN)** is a not-for-profit alliance of leading cancer centers in the United States. Its guidelines are among the most recognized and respected in oncology, providing detailed, evidence-based recommendations for the management of various cancers. The **NCCN Clinical Practice Guidelines in Oncology (NCCN Guidelines)** are updated regularly and incorporate the latest scientific evidence, expert consensus, and real-world clinical experience.

6.1. Key Features of NCCN Guidelines:

1. **Evidence-Based and Continuously Updated**:
   The NCCN guidelines provide recommendations that are grounded in clinical trial data, research findings, and expert consensus. These guidelines are frequently updated to reflect the latest advances in oncology, including new drug approvals, novel therapies, and emerging treatment strategies.
2. **Comprehensive Coverage of Cancer Types**:
   NCCN guidelines cover nearly every major cancer type, including breast, lung, colorectal, prostate, ovarian, and hematologic malignancies like leukemia and lymphoma. For each cancer type, the guidelines provide recommendations for screening, diagnosis, staging, and both initial and follow-up treatments.
3. **Multidisciplinary Approach**:
   The NCCN emphasizes a multidisciplinary approach to cancer care, integrating surgical oncology, radiation oncology, medical oncology, pathology, and supportive care in its treatment recommendations. This reflects the complexity of cancer treatment and the need for collaboration across specialties.
4. **Detailed Treatment Algorithms**:
   For each cancer, the NCCN provides step-by-step treatment algorithms based on cancer stage and patient factors, such as age, comorbidities, and tumor-specific characteristics. These treatment algorithms help guide healthcare providers in selecting the appropriate treatment modality, including surgery, chemotherapy, radiation therapy, immunotherapy, and targeted therapy.
5. **Personalized Medicine**:
   Many NCCN guidelines incorporate molecular and genetic profiling to guide treatment decisions, ensuring that therapies are tailored to individual patients. For example, targeted therapies for **EGFR**, **ALK**, and **ROS1** mutations in non-small cell lung cancer (NSCLC) and **BRCA** mutation testing in breast and ovarian cancers are included in the treatment protocols.
6. **Supportive and Palliative Care**:
   The NCCN also provides comprehensive guidelines for managing cancer-related symptoms and side effects, such as pain, nausea, fatigue, and depression. In addition, they offer palliative care guidelines for improving quality of life in patients with advanced or terminal cancers.

6.2. Breast Cancer

Breast cancer is the most common cancer among women worldwide, and its management has evolved significantly due to advancements in screening, risk stratification, and personalized treatment approaches.

6.2.1. Staging and Risk Stratification in Breast Cancer

Staging breast cancer is a critical step in determining prognosis and treatment. The **TNM system**—assessing **Tumor (T)** size, **Node (N)** involvement, and **Metastasis (M)**—remains the standard for staging breast cancer and is incorporated into both the NCCN and NIH guidelines. The stage of breast cancer significantly influences treatment decisions and prognosis:

- **Stage I**: Small tumors (≤2 cm) with no lymph node involvement.
- **Stage II**: Larger tumors (2-5 cm) or small tumors with limited lymph node involvement.
- **Stage III**: Locally advanced tumors with significant lymph node involvement but no distant metastasis.
- **Stage IV**: Metastatic disease where cancer has spread to distant organs.

In addition to TNM staging, molecular profiling is critical for guiding therapy, particularly in **estrogen receptor-positive (ER+)** breast cancer. For early-stage ER+ breast cancer, **risk stratification tools** like Oncotype DX are commonly used to predict the risk of recurrence and guide chemotherapy decisions.

Oncotype DX Risk Stratification

Oncotype DX is a genomic test that analyzes the expression of 21 genes in the tumor to generate a **recurrence score** (RS). This score helps clinicians determine the benefit of adjuvant chemotherapy in **node-negative**, **ER-positive** breast cancer patients. Based on NIH and NCCN guidelines:

- **Low Recurrence Score (RS ≤ 25)**: Patients with low scores may safely avoid chemotherapy and be treated with hormonal therapy alone. Studies have shown that patients with low RS have excellent outcomes with hormonal therapy alone, with minimal benefit from chemotherapy.
- **High Recurrence Score (RS > 25)**: For patients with high RS, chemotherapy is recommended in addition to hormonal therapy, as studies indicate that chemotherapy significantly reduces the risk of recurrence in this group.

A landmark study, **TAILORx (Trial Assigning IndividuaLized Options for Treatment)**, demonstrated that women with **low-to-intermediate RS** could safely forgo chemotherapy, while those with **high RS** had improved survival when chemotherapy was added to hormonal therapy.

6.2.2. Treatment Options for Breast Cancer

Breast cancer treatment is multimodal and depends on the tumor stage, hormone receptor status, HER2 expression, and patient factors. According to NCCN and NIH guidelines, treatment options include:

Surgery

- **Lumpectomy (Breast-Conserving Surgery)**: This option involves removing the tumor and a margin of surrounding tissue. It is typically followed by **radiation therapy** to minimize the risk of local recurrence. Lumpectomy is often preferred for **early-stage breast cancer** when the tumor size and location are compatible with breast conservation.
- **Mastectomy**: In cases where breast conservation is not possible, such as in **large tumors** or patient preference, mastectomy (removal of the entire breast) is performed. In some cases, mastectomy may be followed by **reconstruction**.
- **Sentinel Lymph Node Biopsy**: This procedure helps determine whether cancer has spread to lymph nodes and is commonly performed with both lumpectomy and mastectomy for staging purposes.

Radiation Therapy

- **Post-Lumpectomy Radiation**: Radiation therapy is standard after lumpectomy to reduce the risk of local recurrence. Studies show that radiation reduces the risk of local recurrence by up to 50%.
- **Post-Mastectomy Radiation**: In cases with large tumors or extensive lymph node involvement, radiation may be recommended after mastectomy to reduce the risk of chest wall recurrence.

Chemotherapy

Chemotherapy is recommended for **higher-stage disease** or when risk stratification tools (like Oncotype DX) suggest a high risk of recurrence. Standard regimens include **AC-T (doxorubicin, cyclophosphamide, paclitaxel)** and **FEC-D (5-fluorouracil, epirubicin, cyclophosphamide, docetaxel)**.

- **Neoadjuvant Chemotherapy**: In some cases, chemotherapy is given **before surgery** to shrink large tumors, making lumpectomy possible or to assess the tumor's response to systemic therapy.

Hormonal Therapy for ER+ Tumors

Hormonal therapy is the cornerstone of treatment for **ER-positive (ER+) breast cancer**, aimed at blocking estrogen signaling to slow or stop tumor growth. The most commonly used hormonal therapies are:

- **Tamoxifen**: A **selective estrogen receptor modulator (SERM)** used in both pre- and postmenopausal women. Tamoxifen has been shown to reduce the risk of recurrence by 50% in ER+ breast cancer patients.
- **Aromatase Inhibitors (AIs)**: These drugs, such as **anastrozole, letrozole**, and **exemestane**, block estrogen production in postmenopausal women. AIs are preferred for postmenopausal women due to their superior efficacy in reducing recurrence compared to tamoxifen.

Targeted Therapy for HER2-Positive Tumors

For **HER2-positive** breast cancer, **HER2-directed therapies** are integral to treatment:

- **Trastuzumab (Herceptin)**: A monoclonal antibody that targets the HER2 receptor, trastuzumab significantly improves outcomes in both early and advanced HER2-positive breast cancer. Studies show that adding trastuzumab to chemotherapy reduces the risk of recurrence by nearly 50%.
- **Pertuzumab (Perjeta)**: Used in combination with trastuzumab, pertuzumab is effective in treating advanced or metastatic HER2-positive breast cancer.
- **Neoadjuvant HER2-Targeted Therapy**: Trastuzumab and pertuzumab are also used in the **neoadjuvant setting** (before surgery) to shrink tumors, improving surgical outcomes.

6.2.3. Latest Advances in Breast Cancer Treatment

The management of breast cancer continues to evolve with the introduction of novel therapies that provide more personalized and effective treatment options. Some of the most recent advances include:

PARP Inhibitors

PARP inhibitors, such as **olaparib**, are a class of drugs that exploit a tumor's defective DNA repair mechanisms, particularly in cancers with **BRCA1/2 mutations**. Olaparib has been approved for use in **BRCA-mutated breast cancer**, particularly in metastatic settings. **OlympiAD**, a clinical trial led by Robson et al. (2017), demonstrated that olaparib significantly improved **progression-free survival (PFS)** in patients with **BRCA-mutated, HER2-negative breast cancer** compared to traditional chemotherapy.

CDK4/6 Inhibitors

For **advanced ER+ breast cancer, CDK4/6 inhibitors** such as **palbociclib, ribociclib**, and **abemaciclib** have shown remarkable efficacy when combined with hormonal therapy (e.g., letrozole or fulvestrant). These drugs work by inhibiting the **cyclin-dependent kinases (CDK4 and CDK6)**, proteins that promote cell cycle progression and cancer cell proliferation.

- **Efficacy**: Clinical trials have shown that adding CDK4/6 inhibitors to hormonal therapy significantly extends **progression-free survival** in patients with advanced or metastatic

ER+ breast cancer. For example, the **MONALEESA-7** trial demonstrated that **ribociclib** combined with hormonal therapy reduced the risk of disease progression by 41% compared to hormonal therapy alone in premenopausal women with advanced breast cancer.

6.3. Lung Cancer

Lung cancer remains one of the leading causes of cancer-related mortality worldwide. It is broadly classified into two major types: **Non-Small Cell Lung Cancer (NSCLC)** and **Small Cell Lung Cancer (SCLC)**, which are treated differently due to variations in biology, growth patterns, and responses to therapy.

6.3.1. Non-Small Cell Lung Cancer (NSCLC)

NSCLC accounts for approximately 85% of all lung cancer cases and includes subtypes such as **adenocarcinoma**, **squamous cell carcinoma**, and **large cell carcinoma**. Treatment is determined by the stage at diagnosis and the molecular characteristics of the tumor.

Early-Stage NSCLC (Stages I-II)

In **early-stage NSCLC**, the primary treatment is **surgery**, which offers the best chance for cure. **Lobectomy** (removal of a lung lobe) is the preferred surgical approach, although **segmentectomy** or **wedge resection** may be used in patients who cannot tolerate a lobectomy due to poor pulmonary function or comorbidities.

- **Adjuvant Therapy**: For patients with **stage II** or high-risk **stage I** disease, **adjuvant chemotherapy** may be recommended to reduce the risk of recurrence. **Platinum-based chemotherapy** (e.g., **cisplatin** combined with **vinorelbine**) has been shown to improve survival in this setting.

Locally Advanced NSCLC (Stage III)

Stage III NSCLC represents a more complex clinical scenario, often requiring a **multimodal approach** that includes **chemotherapy**, **radiation therapy**, and, in some cases, **surgery**.

- **Chemoradiation**: **Concurrent chemoradiation** (the combination of chemotherapy and radiation therapy given simultaneously) is the standard treatment for patients with **unresectable stage III NSCLC**. The combination of chemotherapy (commonly **cisplatin** or **carboplatin** with **etoposide**) and radiation therapy has been shown to improve local control and overall survival.
- **Durvalumab**: For patients who do not progress after chemoradiation, **durvalumab** (a PD-L1 inhibitor) is now standard care based on the **PACIFIC trial**. In this study, patients who received **durvalumab** as **consolidation therapy** following chemoradiation had a significantly longer **progression-free survival (PFS)** and **overall survival (OS)** compared to placebo.

Metastatic NSCLC (Stage IV)

For patients with **metastatic NSCLC**, treatment is driven by **molecular profiling** to identify actionable mutations. Targeted therapies and immunotherapies have revolutionized the management of this stage of the disease.

- **EGFR Mutations**: For patients with **EGFR-mutated NSCLC**, **EGFR tyrosine kinase inhibitors (TKIs)** such as **erlotinib, gefitinib**, and **osimertinib** are the preferred first-line treatments. **Osimertinib** has shown superior efficacy in both **progression-free survival** and **overall survival** compared to earlier-generation EGFR inhibitors, especially in patients with central nervous system metastases.
- **ALK and ROS1 Rearrangements**: Patients with **ALK or ROS1 gene rearrangements** benefit from **ALK inhibitors** like **crizotinib, alectinib,** or **brigatinib. Solomon et al. (2014)** demonstrated that crizotinib significantly improves **progression-free survival** in **ALK-positive NSCLC** compared to chemotherapy, establishing it as the standard treatment for this patient population.
- **PD-L1 Expression and Immunotherapy**: **Immunotherapy** has become a cornerstone of treatment for **advanced NSCLC**. In patients with **high PD-L1 expression (≥50%)**, **checkpoint inhibitors** such as **pembrolizumab** (Keytruda) are used as first-line therapy. In the **KEYNOTE-024 trial, pembrolizumab** monotherapy significantly improved **overall survival** compared to chemotherapy in patients with high PD-L1 expression. For patients with lower PD-L1 expression, immunotherapy is often combined with chemotherapy for improved outcomes.

6.3.2. Small Cell Lung Cancer (SCLC)

SCLC is an aggressive cancer that accounts for approximately 15% of lung cancer cases. It is characterized by rapid growth, early metastasis, and a high response rate to chemotherapy and radiation, but it also has a high rate of relapse.

Limited-Stage SCLC

In **limited-stage SCLC** (disease confined to one hemithorax and amenable to a single radiation field), treatment typically involves a combination of **platinum-based chemotherapy** (cisplatin or carboplatin) and **thoracic radiation therapy**.

- **Concurrent Chemoradiation**: The combination of **cisplatin** or **carboplatin** with **etoposide** is the standard regimen. **Concurrent thoracic radiation** with chemotherapy has been shown to improve survival in limited-stage SCLC.
- **Prophylactic Cranial Irradiation (PCI)**: For patients who achieve a complete response, **prophylactic cranial irradiation (PCI)** is recommended to reduce the risk of brain metastases, which are common in SCLC. Studies have shown that PCI significantly improves overall survival in patients who achieve remission after chemoradiation.

Extensive-Stage SCLC

For **extensive-stage SCLC**, where the disease has spread beyond the thorax, systemic therapy with **platinum-based chemotherapy** remains the cornerstone of treatment.

- **Chemotherapy**: The combination of **cisplatin** or **carboplatin** with **etoposide** is the standard regimen for extensive-stage disease. Although response rates are high, relapse is common, and survival remains poor.
- **Immunotherapy**: Recent advances have introduced **immunotherapy** as part of the treatment for extensive-stage SCLC. The addition of **PD-L1 inhibitors** like **atezolizumab** (Tecentriq) or **durvalumab** (Imfinzi) to chemotherapy has shown promising results. In the **IMpower133 trial**, adding **atezolizumab** to carboplatin and etoposide resulted in a significant improvement in **overall survival** compared to chemotherapy alone. Similarly, the **CASPIAN trial** demonstrated that the addition of **durvalumab** to chemotherapy improved survival in extensive-stage SCLC.

6.3.3. Latest Advances in Lung Cancer Treatment

Immunotherapy in NSCLC and SCLC

The introduction of **immune checkpoint inhibitors**, particularly **PD-1/PD-L1 inhibitors**, has revolutionized the treatment of both **NSCLC** and **SCLC**. These therapies work by blocking the interaction between **PD-1** (a receptor on T cells) and **PD-L1** (a ligand often overexpressed by tumor cells), thereby restoring the immune system's ability to attack cancer cells.

- **NSCLC**: **Pembrolizumab** and **nivolumab** are the leading PD-1 inhibitors used in **advanced NSCLC**. Reck et al. (2016) demonstrated that **pembrolizumab** significantly improved **overall survival** in patients with **PD-L1-positive NSCLC** compared to chemotherapy, establishing it as a first-line treatment in this population.
- **SCLC**: The incorporation of **atezolizumab** and **durvalumab** into the treatment of **extensive-stage SCLC** has extended survival for many patients. These immunotherapies are now standard care in combination with platinum-based chemotherapy for patients with newly diagnosed, extensive-stage disease.

Targeted Therapies for Specific Mutations

- **EGFR, ALK, ROS1, and BRAF Mutations**: Advances in molecular diagnostics have led to the identification of several targetable mutations in NSCLC. Drugs like **osimertinib** for EGFR mutations, **alectinib** for ALK rearrangements, and **vemurafenib** for **BRAF mutations** have shown significant improvements in survival and quality of life for patients with these molecular alterations.

6.4. Colorectal Cancer

Colorectal cancer (CRC) is the third most commonly diagnosed cancer and the second leading cause of cancer-related deaths worldwide. Advances in **screening**, **surgical techniques**, **chemotherapy**, and **immunotherapy** have significantly improved survival rates and outcomes for patients with colorectal cancer.

6.4.1. Screening for Colorectal Cancer

Colorectal cancer screening is essential for early detection and prevention, as most cases of colorectal cancer arise from pre-existing **adenomatous polyps**, which can take 10-15 years to progress into invasive cancer. Screening allows for the detection and removal of these polyps before they become malignant, significantly reducing the incidence of colorectal cancer.

Colonoscopy

Colonoscopy remains the **gold standard** for colorectal cancer screening, offering both diagnostic and therapeutic capabilities. During colonoscopy, polyps can be visualized and removed, preventing their progression to cancer. Colonoscopy has a sensitivity of over 95% for detecting adenomas and is recommended for **average-risk individuals starting at age 45**, according to guidelines from the **American Cancer Society (ACS)** and **National Comprehensive Cancer Network (NCCN)**.

- **Impact on Survival**: Colonoscopy has been shown to reduce **colorectal cancer mortality** by up to 68% in individuals who undergo regular screening. Studies, such as the **National Polyp Study**, have demonstrated that polypectomy during colonoscopy reduces the incidence of colorectal cancer by 76-90%.

Other Screening Modalities

While colonoscopy is the gold standard, other screening methods include:

- **FIT-DNA (Fecal Immunochemical Test-DNA)**: This non-invasive test, also known as **Cologuard**, combines testing for **occult blood** in the stool with the detection of **abnormal DNA** associated with colorectal cancer. FIT-DNA is less invasive but has lower sensitivity for detecting advanced adenomas compared to colonoscopy. The **USPSTF** recommends FIT-DNA every three years for individuals who decline or cannot undergo colonoscopy.
- **CT Colonography (Virtual Colonoscopy)**: This imaging-based screening tool uses **CT scanning** to generate 3D images of the colon. Although CT colonography is non-invasive, it requires bowel preparation and cannot remove polyps. Patients with detected polyps need to undergo a follow-up colonoscopy for removal. It is recommended every five years as an alternative screening option.

Early Detection and Impact

Early detection through screening significantly improves prognosis. When colorectal cancer is detected at an **early stage (stage I)**, the 5-year **survival rate** is over 90%. However, for **late-stage disease (stage IV)**, survival drops to about 14%, highlighting the importance of timely screening and detection.

6.4.2. Treatment Options for Colorectal Cancer

Treatment of colorectal cancer depends on the stage of the disease, and a **multimodal approach** is often necessary, including surgery, chemotherapy, and, in some cases, targeted therapies or immunotherapy.

Surgery

For **localized colorectal cancer** (stages I-III), **surgery** is the primary treatment and is often **curative**. Surgical techniques include:

- **Segmental Resection**: Removal of the tumor along with adjacent lymph nodes. For **rectal cancer**, more specialized procedures like **total mesorectal excision (TME)** are employed to achieve complete resection and reduce recurrence rates.
- **Minimally Invasive Surgery**: Techniques such as **laparoscopic surgery** and **robot-assisted surgery** have been shown to reduce recovery time and postoperative complications while maintaining oncological outcomes similar to open surgery.

Chemotherapy

Adjuvant chemotherapy is typically recommended for patients with **stage III** colorectal cancer and select high-risk **stage II** cases to reduce the risk of recurrence. Standard chemotherapy regimens include:

- **FOLFOX** (5-fluorouracil, leucovorin, oxaliplatin): This regimen is commonly used for patients with **stage III colon cancer**. The addition of oxaliplatin to the backbone of 5-fluorouracil and leucovorin has been shown to improve **disease-free survival (DFS)** by approximately 20%.
- **FOLFIRI** (5-fluorouracil, leucovorin, irinotecan): This regimen is often used in the metastatic setting or for patients who cannot tolerate oxaliplatin. **Irinotecan**, a topoisomerase I inhibitor, is effective in controlling tumor growth and extending survival in advanced disease.
- **CAPOX** (Capecitabine and Oxaliplatin): An alternative to FOLFOX, **CAPOX** uses **capecitabine**, an oral prodrug of 5-fluorouracil, combined with oxaliplatin. Studies have shown similar efficacy to FOLFOX, with the convenience of oral administration.

Targeted Therapies for Advanced Disease

For patients with **metastatic colorectal cancer**, the use of **targeted therapies** in combination with chemotherapy has improved outcomes. Some of the key agents include:

- **Bevacizumab (Avastin)**: An anti-angiogenic agent targeting **VEGF**, bevacizumab inhibits the formation of new blood vessels that tumors need to grow. Studies have shown that adding bevacizumab to chemotherapy improves **overall survival (OS)** and **progression-free survival (PFS)** in patients with metastatic colorectal cancer.

- **EGFR Inhibitors (Cetuximab and Panitumumab)**: These drugs target the **epidermal growth factor receptor (EGFR)** and are effective in patients with **wild-type RAS** tumors. Cetuximab and panitumumab have been shown to improve PFS and OS when added to chemotherapy in patients without **KRAS** or **NRAS** mutations.

6.4.3. Latest Updates in Colorectal Cancer Treatment

Immunotherapy for MSI-H Tumors

Recent advances in **immunotherapy** have had a transformative impact on the treatment of **microsatellite instability-high (MSI-H)** or **mismatch repair-deficient (dMMR)** colorectal cancers. **MSI-H** tumors are characterized by a high mutational burden, making them more susceptible to immune checkpoint inhibitors.

- **Checkpoint Inhibitors**: **Pembrolizumab** (Keytruda) and **nivolumab** (Opdivo) are **PD-1 inhibitors** that have shown remarkable efficacy in patients with **MSI-H colorectal cancer**. In the **KEYNOTE-177 trial**, pembrolizumab significantly improved **progression-free survival** and was associated with fewer side effects compared to chemotherapy in the first-line setting for patients with **MSI-H metastatic colorectal cancer**.
- **Long-Term Survival**: Immunotherapy has become a new standard of care for **MSI-H colorectal cancers**, offering durable responses and improved survival rates in patients who previously had limited options with conventional therapies. **Overman et al. (2018)** showed that **nivolumab**, with or without the addition of **ipilimumab (a CTLA-4 inhibitor)**, resulted in durable responses in patients with metastatic MSI-H colorectal cancer, with some patients achieving long-term disease control.

6.5. Prostate Cancer

Prostate cancer is the second most common cancer in men worldwide, and treatment strategies are largely determined by the stage of disease and risk stratification. Advances in screening, surgical techniques, radiation therapy, and the development of **androgen deprivation therapy (ADT)** and newer hormonal agents have improved outcomes in both localized and metastatic prostate cancer.

6.5.1. Localized Prostate Cancer

Localized prostate cancer refers to cancer that is confined to the prostate gland and has not spread to lymph nodes or distant organs. Treatment options for localized disease depend on a combination of factors, including **prostate-specific antigen (PSA) levels**, **Gleason score**, and **clinical staging (TNM system)**. These factors are used to stratify patients into **low-, intermediate-, and high-risk groups**, guiding treatment decisions.

Active Surveillance

For **low-risk prostate cancer** (low PSA levels, Gleason score ≤6, and limited tumor volume), **active surveillance** is a recommended option. This strategy involves regular monitoring of the cancer through **PSA testing**, **digital rectal exams (DREs)**, and **biopsies** without immediate intervention.

- **Evidence of Safety**: Numerous studies have shown that **active surveillance** is a safe approach for carefully selected men with low-risk prostate cancer. The **ProtecT trial** (Hamdy et al., 2016) demonstrated that **active surveillance** did not result in increased prostate cancer-specific mortality compared to surgery or radiation therapy over a 10-year period, making it a viable option for men who wish to avoid or delay the potential side effects of more invasive treatments.

Surgery (Radical Prostatectomy)

For **intermediate-** and **high-risk localized prostate cancer**, **radical prostatectomy**—the surgical removal of the prostate gland and surrounding tissues—is a common treatment option. This approach offers the potential for a cure, particularly in patients with confined disease.

- **Outcomes**: Studies have shown that **radical prostatectomy** provides excellent long-term outcomes for men with localized prostate cancer, particularly in those with intermediate-risk disease. In a landmark study by **Bill-Axelson et al. (2014)**, men who underwent **radical prostatectomy** had significantly lower **prostate cancer-specific mortality** compared to those managed with watchful waiting.

Radiation Therapy

Radiation therapy is another definitive treatment option for localized prostate cancer. It can be delivered in the form of **external beam radiation therapy (EBRT)** or **brachytherapy (internal radiation)**.

- **External Beam Radiation Therapy (EBRT)**: In this approach, high-energy rays are directed at the prostate from outside the body. Studies have shown that **EBRT** is effective for localized and locally advanced prostate cancer, with 10-year **biochemical recurrence-free survival** rates similar to surgery for appropriately selected patients.
- **Brachytherapy**: This involves the placement of radioactive seeds directly into the prostate tissue. Brachytherapy is often combined with **EBRT** or **androgen deprivation therapy (ADT)** for intermediate- and high-risk disease, improving outcomes. A meta-analysis by **Merrick et al. (2013)** found that brachytherapy combined with EBRT results in better **biochemical control** compared to EBRT alone in men with intermediate- and high-risk prostate cancer.

Combination Therapy for High-Risk Disease

For patients with **high-risk localized prostate cancer**, combining **radiation therapy** with **androgen deprivation therapy (ADT)** has been shown to improve outcomes. A major trial by

Bolla et al. (2010) demonstrated that long-term **ADT** (3 years) combined with **EBRT** significantly improved **overall survival** compared to radiation therapy alone in men with high-risk disease.

6.5.2. Metastatic Prostate Cancer

Metastatic prostate cancer is defined by the spread of cancer beyond the prostate to distant sites, such as bones or lymph nodes. **Androgen deprivation therapy (ADT)** is the cornerstone of treatment for metastatic disease, as prostate cancer is driven by **androgens** (male hormones such as testosterone). By lowering androgen levels or blocking their effects, ADT slows the progression of metastatic prostate cancer.

Androgen Deprivation Therapy (ADT)

ADT can be achieved using **luteinizing hormone-releasing hormone (LHRH) agonists** (e.g., **leuprolide, goserelin**) or **LHRH antagonists** (e.g., **degarelix**), both of which suppress testosterone production by the testes. Alternatively, **orchiectomy** (surgical removal of the testes) can be performed.

- **Efficacy of ADT**: Multiple studies have demonstrated that **ADT** effectively reduces **disease progression** and improves **overall survival** in men with metastatic prostate cancer. However, resistance to ADT eventually develops, leading to a state known as **castration-resistant prostate cancer (CRPC)**, where the cancer continues to grow despite low testosterone levels.

Androgen Receptor Inhibitors

As prostate cancer becomes resistant to traditional ADT, newer agents have been developed to target the **androgen receptor** more effectively. These drugs block the androgen receptor's ability to promote cancer growth, even in the setting of low testosterone levels.

- **Enzalutamide**: An **androgen receptor inhibitor**, **enzalutamide** has been shown to improve survival in patients with **metastatic castration-resistant prostate cancer (mCRPC)**. In the **PREVAIL trial** (Beer et al., 2014), **enzalutamide** improved **overall survival** and **radiographic progression-free survival (rPFS)** compared to placebo in men with chemotherapy-naïve mCRPC.
- **Apalutamide**: Similar to enzalutamide, **apalutamide** is an **androgen receptor antagonist** used in patients with **non-metastatic castration-resistant prostate cancer (nmCRPC)**. The **SPARTAN trial** (Smith et al., 2018) demonstrated that **apalutamide** significantly improved **metastasis-free survival** and delayed the time to metastasis in patients with nmCRPC.

Combination of ADT and Newer Agents

The combination of **ADT** with newer agents such as **enzalutamide, apalutamide,** or **abiraterone** (a CYP17 inhibitor that blocks androgen synthesis) is now the standard of care for men with **high-risk non-metastatic** or **metastatic prostate cancer**.

- **Abiraterone**: In the **LATITUDE trial**, the combination of **abiraterone** with ADT improved **overall survival** and delayed disease progression in men with newly diagnosed **high-risk metastatic prostate cancer** compared to ADT alone (Fizazi et al., 2017).

6.5.3. Latest Updates in Prostate Cancer Treatment

Enzalutamide and Apalutamide in CRPC

For patients with **castration-resistant prostate cancer (CRPC)**, newer androgen receptor inhibitors such as **enzalutamide** and **apalutamide** have become integral parts of the treatment paradigm. These agents target androgen signaling more effectively, even in cases where the cancer has progressed despite traditional ADT.

- **Enzalutamide**: In the **PREVAIL** and **AFFIRM** trials, enzalutamide improved **overall survival** and delayed disease progression in men with mCRPC, whether or not they had received previous chemotherapy.
- **Apalutamide**: In the **SPARTAN trial**, apalutamide was shown to significantly prolong **metastasis-free survival** in men with **non-metastatic CRPC**, delaying the onset of metastatic disease.

PARP Inhibitors for DNA-Repair Deficient Prostate Cancer

Recent advances have introduced **PARP inhibitors**, such as **olaparib**, as an option for men with **metastatic CRPC** who harbor mutations in DNA repair genes (e.g., **BRCA1/2**). The **PROfound trial** demonstrated that **olaparib** significantly improved **progression-free survival** and **overall survival** in men with these mutations compared to standard treatment (de Bono et al., 2020).

6.6. Cervical Cancer

Cervical cancer remains a significant global health burden, particularly in low- and middle-income countries where screening programs and access to preventive measures are less prevalent. Advances in **screening, vaccination,** and **treatment strategies**, including the incorporation of **immunotherapy** for advanced disease, have significantly improved outcomes.

6.6.1. Screening for Cervical Cancer

Screening for cervical cancer has led to a significant decline in the incidence and mortality of the disease, particularly in countries with well-established screening programs. Early detection through screening allows for the identification and treatment of **precancerous lesions** (cervical intraepithelial neoplasia), preventing progression to invasive cancer.

Pap Smear (Cytology)

The **Pap smear**, or **Papanicolaou test**, remains a cornerstone of cervical cancer screening. The test involves the collection of cervical cells, which are then examined under a microscope for precancerous or cancerous changes.

- **Effectiveness**: Studies have shown that regular **Pap smear screening** reduces cervical cancer incidence by up to 80% in women who are screened regularly. The **U.S. Preventive Services Task Force (USPSTF)** recommends **Pap smears** every **three years** for women aged **21-65**.

HPV Testing

Human papillomavirus (HPV) testing has emerged as a complementary and, in some cases, alternative approach to cytology-based screening. **HPV infection**, particularly with **high-risk types (HPV 16 and 18)**, is the primary cause of cervical cancer, and testing for the presence of high-risk HPV strains is an important tool in identifying women at increased risk of cervical cancer.

- **Combined Pap and HPV Testing (Co-testing)**: For women aged **30-65**, the **USPSTF** recommends either **co-testing** with **Pap smears and HPV testing every five years** or Pap smears alone every three years. Studies have shown that **HPV testing** is more sensitive than cytology alone for detecting high-grade cervical lesions.

HPV Vaccination

The development and widespread implementation of the **HPV vaccine** has been one of the most significant public health advances in the prevention of cervical cancer. Vaccination against high-risk HPV types (particularly HPV 16 and 18) has been shown to dramatically reduce the incidence of **HPV-related cervical lesions** and **cervical cancer**.

- **Vaccine Efficacy**: **Long-term studies** have demonstrated that the **quadrivalent (Gardasil)** and **nonavalent (Gardasil 9)** vaccines offer robust protection against persistent HPV infection and cervical intraepithelial neoplasia (CIN). A **2017 study** published in **The Lancet** confirmed that HPV vaccination led to a **70% reduction** in the incidence of high-grade cervical lesions in vaccinated cohorts.
- **Vaccination Guidelines**: The **Centers for Disease Control and Prevention (CDC)** recommends routine vaccination for boys and girls at ages **11-12**, with catch-up vaccination available through age 26 for those who missed earlier vaccination opportunities.

6.6.2. Treatment Options for Cervical Cancer

The treatment of cervical cancer depends on the **stage of the disease**, with options ranging from surgery for early-stage disease to **chemoradiation** for locally advanced disease.

Advanced or metastatic cervical cancer often requires systemic therapy, and recent advances in **immunotherapy** have provided new treatment options for these patients.

Surgical Options for Early-Stage Cervical Cancer

For patients with **early-stage cervical cancer** (stage I and select stage II disease), **surgery** remains the standard curative option.

- **Hysterectomy**: The most common surgical approach for early-stage cervical cancer is **radical hysterectomy**, which involves the removal of the uterus, cervix, part of the vagina, and surrounding tissues. For small, early tumors, **simple hysterectomy** (removal of the uterus and cervix without extensive tissue removal) may be sufficient.
- **Fertility-Preserving Surgery**: For women who wish to preserve fertility and have **very early-stage disease (stage IA)**, **conization** (removal of a cone-shaped piece of the cervix) or **radical trachelectomy** (removal of the cervix while preserving the uterus) may be considered. Studies have shown that these approaches can safely preserve fertility in select patients with early-stage cervical cancer.

Chemoradiation for Locally Advanced Cervical Cancer

For patients with **locally advanced cervical cancer** (stage IIb-IVa), the standard treatment is **chemoradiation**, which combines **external beam radiation therapy (EBRT)** and **brachytherapy** with concurrent **platinum-based chemotherapy** (usually **cisplatin**).

- **Effectiveness of Chemoradiation**: Multiple randomized trials, including a **meta-analysis by Chemoradiotherapy for Cervical Cancer Meta-analysis Collaboration (CCCMAC, 2010)**, have demonstrated that **concurrent chemoradiation** improves **overall survival (OS)** and **progression-free survival (PFS)** compared to radiation alone. **Cisplatin-based chemoradiation** has become the gold standard for the treatment of **locally advanced cervical cancer**.
- **Brachytherapy**: The use of **intracavitary brachytherapy** as part of the radiation regimen is essential for controlling the tumor and improving survival outcomes in locally advanced disease. Studies have shown that **brachytherapy** in combination with EBRT improves local control and decreases the risk of recurrence.

6.6.3. Latest Advances in Cervical Cancer Treatment

Recent advances in systemic therapies, particularly **immunotherapy**, have provided new hope for patients with **advanced** or **recurrent cervical cancer**, where options were previously limited.

Immunotherapy for Advanced Cervical Cancer

The introduction of **immune checkpoint inhibitors** has revolutionized the treatment landscape for several cancers, including cervical cancer. **Pembrolizumab** is a **PD-1 inhibitor** that has shown promising results in patients with advanced or recurrent cervical cancer, particularly those expressing **PD-L1** on their tumors.

- **Approval of Pembrolizumab**: Based on the results of the **KEYNOTE-158 trial**, the **FDA** approved **pembrolizumab** for patients with **PD-L1-positive recurrent or metastatic cervical cancer** who have progressed on chemotherapy. In this study, pembrolizumab demonstrated **durable responses** in patients with PD-L1-positive tumors, leading to an **overall response rate (ORR)** of 14.6%. Patients who responded to pembrolizumab experienced significant improvements in both **PFS** and **OS** compared to historical controls.

Targeted Therapy for Advanced Cervical Cancer

Recent studies have explored the use of **targeted therapies** in advanced cervical cancer, particularly drugs that target specific molecular pathways involved in tumor growth and angiogenesis.

- **Bevacizumab**: Bevacizumab, an anti-angiogenic agent targeting **vascular endothelial growth factor (VEGF)**, has been shown to improve outcomes in combination with chemotherapy for patients with advanced cervical cancer. The **GOG-240 trial** demonstrated that adding **bevacizumab** to **platinum-based chemotherapy** improved **overall survival** and **response rates** in patients with recurrent, persistent, or metastatic cervical cancer.

6.7. Ovarian Cancer

Ovarian cancer remains one of the deadliest gynecologic cancers, primarily due to its asymptomatic nature in early stages and lack of effective screening methods for the general population. Most patients are diagnosed at an advanced stage, where the prognosis is poorer. However, advancements in treatment, particularly with targeted therapies and maintenance strategies, have improved outcomes for many patients.

6.7.1. Screening for Ovarian Cancer

Unlike other cancers such as breast or cervical cancer, there is **no effective screening test** for ovarian cancer in the general population. Both **NCCN** and **USPSTF** recommend against routine screening in asymptomatic women at average risk due to the lack of demonstrated benefit in reducing mortality.

High-Risk Populations

For women at **high risk**, such as those with **BRCA1/2 mutations** or **Lynch syndrome** (hereditary non-polyposis colorectal cancer), risk-reduction strategies are different. These women may benefit from:

- **Genetic Testing and Counseling**: Women with a strong family history of ovarian or breast cancer should be referred for **genetic counseling** to assess for mutations in **BRCA1**, **BRCA2**, or other related genes.
- **Risk-Reducing Surgery**: Prophylactic **bilateral salpingo-oophorectomy** (removal of the ovaries and fallopian tubes) is the most effective strategy for reducing ovarian cancer risk in BRCA mutation carriers.
- **Surveillance**: While there is no proven effective screening for high-risk women, some guidelines suggest regular **transvaginal ultrasound** and **CA-125 blood tests** as part of a surveillance program, although evidence supporting their efficacy remains limited.

Lack of Routine Screening for the General Population

Current evidence, including results from the **PLCO (Prostate, Lung, Colorectal, and Ovarian) Cancer Screening Trial**, shows that **CA-125 blood tests** and **transvaginal ultrasound** are not effective in reducing ovarian cancer mortality in average-risk women. These tools often lead to false positives and unnecessary surgeries without improving outcomes.

6.7.2. Treatment of Ovarian Cancer: NCCN Guidelines

The **NCCN guidelines** provide a comprehensive framework for treating ovarian cancer, focusing on a multimodal approach that includes **surgery**, **chemotherapy**, and **targeted therapies**. The treatment varies based on disease stage, molecular profile, and patient characteristics.

Surgery (Cytoreductive Surgery)

Cytoreductive surgery (also known as debulking surgery) is the cornerstone of treatment for most patients with newly diagnosed ovarian cancer. The goal is to remove as much visible tumor as possible, as this is strongly associated with improved survival outcomes.

- **Optimal Cytoreduction**: Optimal surgery, defined as leaving no visible residual tumor, has been shown to significantly improve overall survival. A **meta-analysis** of cytoreductive surgery studies indicated that **optimal cytoreduction** results in better outcomes compared to suboptimal debulking.
- **Neoadjuvant Chemotherapy (NACT)**: For patients with **advanced-stage disease** (stages III-IV) who are not candidates for primary debulking surgery, **neoadjuvant chemotherapy (NACT)** followed by **interval debulking surgery (IDS)** is an alternative. The **CHORUS trial** demonstrated that **NACT** followed by surgery achieved similar outcomes to primary surgery with fewer surgical complications.

Chemotherapy

Postoperative chemotherapy is standard for most patients with ovarian cancer, particularly those with advanced-stage disease.

- **Platinum-Based Chemotherapy**: The standard regimen is a combination of **carboplatin** and **paclitaxel**. These agents have demonstrated significant efficacy in improving **progression-free survival (PFS)** and **overall survival (OS)** in women with advanced ovarian cancer.
- **Intraperitoneal (IP) Chemotherapy**: For select patients with optimally debulked disease, **intraperitoneal chemotherapy** (directly delivering chemotherapy into the peritoneal cavity) has shown improved survival. The **GOG-172 trial** demonstrated better survival outcomes with IP chemotherapy compared to IV chemotherapy alone, but its use has declined due to increased toxicity and logistical challenges.

6.7.3. Latest Advances in Ovarian Cancer Treatment

Recent advancements in ovarian cancer treatment focus on **PARP inhibitors** and **anti-angiogenic agents**, which have changed the treatment landscape, especially in patients with BRCA mutations or recurrent disease.

PARP Inhibitors

PARP inhibitors are a major breakthrough in the treatment of **BRCA-mutated ovarian cancer**. They exploit the concept of **synthetic lethality** by inhibiting PARP, an enzyme involved in DNA repair, leading to cancer cell death in tumors with defective **BRCA-mediated homologous recombination repair**.

- **Olaparib**: Olaparib was the first PARP inhibitor approved for the treatment of recurrent **BRCA-mutated ovarian cancer**. Recent data from the **SOLO-1 trial** demonstrated that olaparib as **maintenance therapy** after first-line platinum-based chemotherapy significantly improves **PFS** in patients with **BRCA mutations**. The study reported a **70% reduction** in the risk of progression or death with olaparib, making it a game-changer for these patients.
- **Other PARP Inhibitors**: Additional PARP inhibitors like **niraparib** and **rucaparib** are also used in both BRCA-mutated and **homologous recombination deficiency (HRD)-**positive ovarian cancers. The **PRIMA trial** showed that **niraparib**, as maintenance therapy in patients with advanced ovarian cancer, improved PFS, regardless of BRCA mutation status.

Bevacizumab (Anti-Angiogenic Therapy)

Bevacizumab is an **anti-angiogenic agent** that targets **vascular endothelial growth factor (VEGF)**, reducing the blood supply to tumors. It has been approved for use in combination with chemotherapy in patients with **advanced-stage ovarian cancer**.

- **GOG-0218 Trial**: In the **GOG-0218 trial**, the addition of **bevacizumab** to standard platinum-based chemotherapy followed by **bevacizumab maintenance** significantly improved **progression-free survival** in patients with advanced ovarian cancer. This

established **bevacizumab** as an important component of frontline therapy, particularly in patients with high-risk disease.
- **Recurrent Disease**: In the recurrent setting, the **AURELIA trial** demonstrated that adding **bevacizumab** to chemotherapy improved **response rates** and **PFS** in patients with platinum-resistant ovarian cancer.

Maintenance Therapy

For patients who respond to platinum-based chemotherapy, **maintenance therapy** with PARP inhibitors or bevacizumab has become a standard of care to delay recurrence and prolong survival.

- **Olaparib**: As demonstrated in the **SOLO-1 trial**, olaparib maintenance therapy significantly extended PFS in newly diagnosed patients with **BRCA-mutated ovarian cancer**, with ongoing studies evaluating the long-term impact on overall survival.
- **Niraparib**: The **PRIMA trial** showed that **niraparib** maintenance therapy provided a **progression-free survival benefit** in both BRCA-mutated and BRCA wild-type patients, offering a broader application of PARP inhibition beyond just BRCA-mutated cancers.

6.8. Pancreatic Cancer

Pancreatic cancer is one of the most aggressive and deadly cancers, with a five-year survival rate of less than 10%. Due to its late-stage diagnosis, often after symptoms have developed, pancreatic cancer remains challenging to treat. Significant advances have been made in the areas of **surgical techniques**, **chemotherapy regimens**, and **targeted therapies**, improving outcomes for some patients.

6.8.1. Screening for Pancreatic Cancer

Pancreatic cancer screening is not routinely recommended for the general population due to its low prevalence and the lack of an effective, non-invasive screening test. Screening is generally reserved for **high-risk individuals** who have a significantly increased risk of developing pancreatic cancer, including those with a strong family history of the disease or known genetic mutations.

Screening in High-Risk Populations

For individuals with **hereditary cancer syndromes** or a strong family history of pancreatic cancer, **NCCN guidelines** recommend surveillance with **endoscopic ultrasound (EUS)** and **magnetic resonance imaging (MRI)** or **MR cholangiopancreatography (MRCP)**.

- **Hereditary Syndromes**: Individuals with hereditary syndromes such as **BRCA1/2 mutations, Lynch syndrome, Peutz-Jeghers syndrome**, or **familial pancreatic cancer (FPC)** are considered at high risk. Genetic testing for these mutations, particularly in those with a strong family history of pancreatic or other cancers, is recommended.

- **Screening Modalities**: EUS and MRI/MRCP are preferred modalities because they are non-invasive and have higher sensitivity for detecting early pancreatic abnormalities or intraductal papillary mucinous neoplasms (IPMNs), which can be precursors to pancreatic cancer. These tests are typically performed annually in high-risk individuals.

Lack of Routine Screening in the General Population

There are currently no validated blood tests or imaging techniques that are sensitive and specific enough to screen the general population for pancreatic cancer. Biomarkers such as **CA 19-9** are sometimes used to monitor disease in patients already diagnosed with pancreatic cancer but are not effective for early detection in asymptomatic individuals.

6.8.2. Treatment of Pancreatic Cancer: NCCN Guidelines

The treatment of pancreatic cancer depends on the **stage of disease** at diagnosis and whether the tumor is deemed **resectable, borderline resectable**, or **unresectable/metastatic**. The primary modalities for treatment include **surgery, chemotherapy**, and **radiation therapy**, with **NCCN guidelines** emphasizing a **multidisciplinary approach** for optimal outcomes.

Surgical Treatment for Resectable and Borderline Resectable Disease

For patients with **resectable** pancreatic cancer (approximately 15-20% of cases at diagnosis), surgery offers the best chance for long-term survival. However, even with successful resection, recurrence rates are high, and most patients will require adjuvant chemotherapy.

- **Pancreaticoduodenectomy (Whipple Procedure)**: The **Whipple procedure** is the most common surgery for tumors in the **head of the pancreas**. It involves removal of the head of the pancreas, parts of the small intestine, bile duct, and sometimes part of the stomach.
- **Distal Pancreatectomy**: For tumors located in the **body or tail of the pancreas**, a **distal pancreatectomy** is performed, often along with a splenectomy.
- **Evidence of Improved Outcomes**: A retrospective study by **Katz et al. (2008)** demonstrated that patients with **borderline resectable pancreatic cancer** who underwent **neoadjuvant chemotherapy** followed by surgery had significantly improved **overall survival (OS)** compared to those who had immediate surgery. This supports the use of neoadjuvant therapy in this population to increase the likelihood of complete resection.

Neoadjuvant Therapy for Borderline Resectable Disease

For **borderline resectable pancreatic cancer**, **neoadjuvant therapy** (chemotherapy ± radiation) is often recommended before surgery. This approach may shrink the tumor, making surgical resection more likely, and also helps to treat micrometastatic disease early.

- **FOLFIRINOX and Gemcitabine-Based Regimens**: FOLFIRINOX (a combination of 5-fluorouracil, leucovorin, irinotecan, and oxaliplatin) is a common neoadjuvant chemotherapy regimen used for fit patients. Studies, such as **PREOPANC**, have shown that neoadjuvant therapy increases the likelihood of achieving an **R0 resection** (no residual tumor) and improves **overall survival** compared to immediate surgery.

Adjuvant Chemotherapy

For patients with resected pancreatic cancer, **adjuvant chemotherapy** is the standard of care to reduce the risk of recurrence. **Gemcitabine** and **FOLFIRINOX** are the most commonly used regimens.

- **ESPAC-4 Trial**: The **ESPAC-4 trial** demonstrated that **adjuvant gemcitabine plus capecitabine** improved **overall survival** compared to gemcitabine alone in patients with resected pancreatic cancer. The median survival in the combination therapy group was **28 months**, compared to **25.5 months** with gemcitabine alone.
- **PRODIGE 24/CCTG PA.6 Trial**: The **PRODIGE 24** trial established **modified FOLFIRINOX** as the new standard for adjuvant chemotherapy in fit patients with resected pancreatic cancer. The trial showed a significant improvement in **overall survival** (median OS of **54.4 months** with FOLFIRINOX vs. **35 months** with gemcitabine).

6.8.3. Treatment of Unresectable and Metastatic Disease

For patients with **unresectable** or **metastatic pancreatic cancer**, treatment is focused on systemic therapy to prolong survival and palliate symptoms.

Systemic Chemotherapy

- **FOLFIRINOX**: In the **metastatic setting**, FOLFIRINOX has been shown to significantly improve **overall survival** and **progression-free survival (PFS)** compared to gemcitabine. The **ACCORD-11 trial** reported a median OS of **11.1 months** for patients treated with **FOLFIRINOX** versus **6.8 months** for gemcitabine alone.
- **Gemcitabine Plus Nab-Paclitaxel**: Another commonly used regimen in **unresectable or metastatic disease** is **gemcitabine plus nab-paclitaxel**. The **MPACT trial** showed that this combination improved median OS (8.5 months vs. 6.7 months with gemcitabine alone) in patients with metastatic pancreatic cancer.

Targeted Therapy and Immunotherapy

Targeted therapies and **immunotherapies** have shown limited efficacy in pancreatic cancer, but recent advances in understanding the molecular biology of the disease have opened the door for new approaches.

- **PARP Inhibitors (Olaparib)**: For patients with **BRCA1/2 mutations** (which are present in a small percentage of pancreatic cancer patients), **PARP inhibitors** like **olaparib** have shown promise. The **POLO trial** demonstrated that **olaparib** as maintenance therapy improved **progression-free survival** in patients with **germline BRCA-mutated**

metastatic pancreatic cancer who had responded to first-line platinum-based chemotherapy.
- **Immunotherapy (Checkpoint Inhibitors)**: While most pancreatic cancers do not respond to **immune checkpoint inhibitors**, a small subset of patients with **microsatellite instability-high (MSI-H)** tumors may benefit from **pembrolizumab**. The **KEYNOTE-158 trial** showed durable responses in patients with MSI-H pancreatic cancer, leading to **FDA approval** of pembrolizumab for this biomarker-positive subset.

6.8.4. Latest Advances in Pancreatic Cancer Treatment

PARP Inhibitors

The use of **PARP inhibitors** like **olaparib** in patients with **BRCA1/2 mutations** represents a significant advance in the personalized treatment of pancreatic cancer. The **POLO trial** showed that maintenance therapy with olaparib improved **progression-free survival** by more than three months compared to placebo, offering a targeted treatment option for this select group of patients.

Immune Checkpoint Inhibitors

While **immune checkpoint inhibitors** have not broadly transformed pancreatic cancer treatment, ongoing research is investigating combination strategies to enhance immune responses. Trials combining **checkpoint inhibitors** with **chemotherapy** or **targeted therapies** are being explored to overcome the immune-resistant nature of pancreatic tumors.

Tumor Microenvironment Targeting

Pancreatic cancer's **desmoplastic stroma** is a dense fibrous tissue that creates a barrier to effective drug delivery. Research efforts are ongoing to target the **tumor microenvironment**, including the development of agents that can disrupt the stroma or enhance drug penetration.

6.9. Bladder Cancer

Bladder cancer is the fourth most common cancer in men and ninth in women, with **urothelial carcinoma** being the most common histologic subtype. The management of bladder cancer has advanced significantly in recent years, particularly in the realms of **immunotherapy**, **targeted therapies**, and **enhanced surgical techniques**.

6.9.1. Screening for Bladder Cancer

Routine screening for bladder cancer in the general population is **not recommended** due to the absence of a proven mortality benefit. Screening is typically considered only in specific high-risk populations, such as individuals with a significant smoking history or occupational exposure to bladder carcinogens (e.g., in the chemical or dye industry).

Screening for High-Risk Populations

For patients at high risk, screening may involve regular surveillance through **urinalysis**, **urine cytology**, or **urinary biomarkers**. These patients include:

- **Long-term smokers**: Smoking is the most significant risk factor for bladder cancer, accounting for nearly 50% of all cases.
- **Occupational exposure**: Workers in industries involving chemicals such as aromatic amines, dyes, rubber, or leather production are at increased risk.
- **Prior history of bladder cancer**: Patients who have previously been treated for bladder cancer require regular surveillance due to high recurrence rates.

Urinary Biomarkers

While urinary biomarkers, such as **NMP22** (nuclear matrix protein 22) and **Bladder Tumor Antigen (BTA)**, have been investigated for their utility in detecting bladder cancer, they are not yet part of routine screening due to limitations in specificity and sensitivity.

6.9.2. Treatment of Bladder Cancer: NCCN Guidelines

The **NCCN guidelines** for bladder cancer stratify treatment recommendations based on the clinical stage of the disease, distinguishing between **non-muscle-invasive bladder cancer (NMIBC)**, **muscle-invasive bladder cancer (MIBC)**, and **metastatic disease**. Treatment modalities include **surgery**, **intravesical therapy**, **systemic chemotherapy**, **radiation**, and **immunotherapy**.

Non-Muscle-Invasive Bladder Cancer (NMIBC)

For patients with NMIBC (stages **Ta**, **T1**, and **CIS**), the primary treatment goal is to remove visible tumors and prevent recurrence or progression.

- **Transurethral Resection of Bladder Tumor (TURBT)**: TURBT is the first-line treatment for NMIBC, allowing for the removal of visible tumors and precise staging of the disease. Following TURBT, patients are typically stratified into **low-risk**, **intermediate-risk**, or **high-risk** groups based on tumor grade, size, and recurrence risk.
- **Intravesical Therapy**: Patients with **intermediate-** or **high-risk NMIBC** benefit from **intravesical therapy**, which is delivered directly into the bladder to reduce the risk of recurrence and progression. Common options include:
  - **Bacillus Calmette-Guerin (BCG)**: The most effective intravesical treatment, BCG has been shown to reduce both tumor recurrence and progression. The **SWOG 8507 trial** demonstrated that maintenance BCG therapy significantly improves **disease-free survival** compared to induction therapy alone.
  - **Intravesical Chemotherapy**: Agents such as **mitomycin C** or **gemcitabine** are alternatives to BCG, particularly in patients who cannot tolerate or do not respond to BCG. The **BRIDGE trial** demonstrated that intravesical gemcitabine is effective for BCG-refractory NMIBC, with a lower toxicity profile.

Muscle-Invasive Bladder Cancer (MIBC)

For patients with **muscle-invasive bladder cancer (stage T2 or greater)**, treatment typically involves a **multimodal approach** combining surgery, chemotherapy, and, in some cases, radiation.

- **Radical Cystectomy**: **Radical cystectomy** (removal of the bladder, surrounding tissues, and regional lymph nodes) is the gold standard for **muscle-invasive bladder cancer**. In patients who are candidates for surgery, it offers the best chance for cure. The NCCN guidelines recommend radical cystectomy with pelvic lymph node dissection as the preferred treatment for localized MIBC.
- **Neoadjuvant Chemotherapy**: The addition of **neoadjuvant chemotherapy** before surgery has been shown to improve **overall survival (OS)**. The most commonly used regimen is **cisplatin-based combination therapy**, such as **MVAC** (methotrexate, vinblastine, doxorubicin, cisplatin) or **gemcitabine-cisplatin**. The landmark **ABC meta-analysis** demonstrated that neoadjuvant chemotherapy improved **5-year overall survival** by 5-10%.
- **Bladder-Sparing Approaches**: For patients who are not candidates for radical cystectomy, **bladder-sparing protocols** using a combination of **chemoradiation** may be an alternative. Studies such as the **RTOG 8903 trial** have shown that chemoradiation can achieve comparable local control and survival rates to surgery in selected patients.

Metastatic Bladder Cancer

For patients with **metastatic bladder cancer** (stage IV), the primary treatment goal is to prolong survival and palliate symptoms. The mainstay of treatment for metastatic disease is **systemic chemotherapy**.

- **Cisplatin-Based Chemotherapy**: For patients eligible for platinum-based chemotherapy, the combination of **cisplatin** and **gemcitabine** is the most commonly used regimen, providing improved **overall survival** compared to non-cisplatin regimens. The **EORTC 30987 trial** demonstrated that **gemcitabine/cisplatin** had similar efficacy to **MVAC**, but with a better toxicity profile.
- **Immunotherapy for Platinum-Ineligible Patients**: Patients who cannot receive platinum-based chemotherapy may benefit from **immune checkpoint inhibitors**. **Atezolizumab** and **pembrolizumab**, both **PD-1/PD-L1 inhibitors**, are approved for the treatment of **platinum-ineligible metastatic bladder cancer** based on trials showing durable responses and improved survival. In the **KEYNOTE-045 trial**, **pembrolizumab** improved **overall survival** compared to chemotherapy in patients with platinum-refractory bladder cancer.

6.9.3. Latest Advances in Bladder Cancer Treatment

The treatment landscape for bladder cancer has expanded significantly with the introduction of **immunotherapy**, **targeted therapies**, and novel combinations of therapies.

Immunotherapy for Advanced Bladder Cancer

Immunotherapy has become an integral part of the treatment for advanced bladder cancer, particularly for patients with **metastatic or platinum-refractory disease**.

- **PD-1/PD-L1 Inhibitors**: **Pembrolizumab** (a PD-1 inhibitor) and **atezolizumab** (a PD-L1 inhibitor) have demonstrated durable responses and survival benefits in patients with advanced bladder cancer. In the **KEYNOTE-045 trial**, **pembrolizumab** improved **overall survival** (10.3 months vs. 7.4 months) compared to chemotherapy, establishing it as the preferred second-line therapy after platinum-based chemotherapy.
- **Maintenance Avelumab**: Recent data from the **JAVELIN Bladder 100 trial** introduced the concept of **maintenance immunotherapy**. In this trial, **avelumab**, a PD-L1 inhibitor, was given as **maintenance therapy** after chemotherapy in patients with metastatic urothelial carcinoma who had responded to or stabilized with chemotherapy. The trial demonstrated a significant improvement in **overall survival**, with a median OS of **21.4 months** in the avelumab group compared to **14.3 months** in the control group.

Targeted Therapy

For patients with **FGFR3 mutations**, a subset of patients with advanced bladder cancer can benefit from **FGFR inhibitors**.

- **Erdafitinib**: Erdafitinib is an **FGFR inhibitor** approved for patients with **locally advanced** or **metastatic urothelial carcinoma** harboring FGFR3 or FGFR2 mutations. The **BLC2001 trial** demonstrated that **erdafitinib** produced an **overall response rate (ORR)** of 40% in patients with FGFR mutations, representing a novel option for this specific molecular subtype of bladder cancer.

6.10. Kidney Cancer

Kidney cancer, also known as **renal cell carcinoma (RCC)**, accounts for about 90% of kidney malignancies. It is one of the 10 most common cancers, particularly in men. Over the past decade, there have been significant advancements in the treatment of kidney cancer, with the advent of targeted therapies and immunotherapies revolutionizing patient outcomes.

6.10.1. Screening for Kidney Cancer

There are **no routine screening tests** recommended for the general population to detect kidney cancer. Most kidney cancers are detected incidentally on imaging studies (e.g., ultrasound, CT scan, MRI) performed for unrelated reasons. Early detection typically occurs when the cancer is found at a localized stage, and the prognosis is favorable.

Screening for High-Risk Populations

Although routine screening is not recommended for the general population, certain **high-risk groups** may benefit from surveillance. High-risk individuals include those with **hereditary syndromes** and **strong family histories** of kidney cancer.

- **Von Hippel-Lindau (VHL) Disease**: Patients with **VHL disease**, a genetic condition that predisposes individuals to develop RCC and other tumors, are considered at high risk. The **NCCN guidelines** recommend annual **abdominal imaging (MRI or CT)** for these patients, starting in early adulthood.
- **Hereditary Leiomyomatosis and Renal Cell Cancer (HLRCC)**: Patients with HLRCC have an increased risk of aggressive RCC. Regular surveillance with imaging is recommended.

Incidental Findings

Most kidney cancers are detected incidentally during imaging performed for unrelated reasons. Studies have shown that up to **60% of kidney cancers** are discovered incidentally, and these cases tend to have better outcomes since they are more likely to be localized at the time of diagnosis.

6.10.2. Treatment of Kidney Cancer: NCCN Guidelines

The **NCCN guidelines** stratify kidney cancer treatment based on the stage of the disease and risk factors for recurrence. Treatment options include **surgery**, **systemic therapies** (including targeted therapies and immunotherapies), and **radiation therapy** in certain settings. The choice of treatment depends on the **tumor size**, **stage**, and **histologic subtype**.

Localized Disease (Stage I-III)

For patients with **localized kidney cancer** (stages I-III), the mainstay of treatment is **surgical resection**, with the intent to cure.

- **Partial Nephrectomy**: For **small renal masses (T1 tumors, <7 cm)**, **partial nephrectomy** (nephron-sparing surgery) is preferred over radical nephrectomy to preserve kidney function, especially in patients with pre-existing renal impairment. Studies such as those by **Van Poppel et al. (2011)** showed that partial nephrectomy offers comparable oncologic outcomes to radical nephrectomy for small tumors, with the added benefit of preserving renal function.
- **Radical Nephrectomy**: For larger or more advanced tumors, a **radical nephrectomy** (removal of the kidney, perinephric fat, and sometimes regional lymph nodes) is recommended. **NCCN guidelines** suggest radical nephrectomy for **T2 tumors (>7 cm)** or when the tumor is not amenable to nephron-sparing surgery.
- **Active Surveillance**: In select patients with small, asymptomatic tumors (especially elderly or comorbid patients), **active surveillance** with regular imaging may be an option. **Kunkle et al. (2008)** demonstrated that active surveillance can be a safe option for certain small renal masses, with low rates of progression over time.

Advanced or Metastatic Disease (Stage IV)

For patients with **metastatic renal cell carcinoma (mRCC)**, the treatment paradigm has shifted significantly with the development of **targeted therapies** and **immunotherapies**.

- **Cytoreductive Nephrectomy**: While nephrectomy is typically curative for localized disease, in **metastatic RCC**, cytoreductive nephrectomy (removal of the primary tumor) may still be considered in select patients to improve systemic therapy outcomes. The **CARMENA trial (2018)**, however, showed that **sunitinib alone** was non-inferior to nephrectomy followed by sunitinib in patients with intermediate- or poor-risk mRCC, suggesting that systemic therapy alone may be appropriate for many patients.
- **Systemic Therapy**: The standard of care for **metastatic RCC** involves **targeted therapies** or **immunotherapy**. Historically, **tyrosine kinase inhibitors (TKIs)** targeting the **VEGF** pathway were the backbone of treatment, but **immune checkpoint inhibitors** (ICIs) have now emerged as a major component of therapy.
    - **VEGF-Targeted Therapy (TKIs)**: Agents such as **sunitinib** and **pazopanib** have been mainstays in the treatment of mRCC. The **COMPARZ trial** compared **pazopanib** and **sunitinib** in metastatic RCC and showed that they had similar efficacy, but pazopanib had a better tolerability profile in terms of patient-reported quality of life.
    - **Checkpoint Inhibitors**: Immune checkpoint inhibitors like **nivolumab** (anti-PD-1) and **ipilimumab** (anti-CTLA-4) have changed the treatment landscape for advanced RCC. The **CheckMate 214 trial** demonstrated that the combination of **nivolumab** and **ipilimumab** significantly improved **overall survival (OS)** and **progression-free survival (PFS)** compared to sunitinib in patients with intermediate- and poor-risk mRCC, leading to its approval as a frontline treatment for these patients.
    - **Combination Therapy**: Recent trials have focused on combining **immunotherapy** with **TKIs**. The **KEYNOTE-426 trial** demonstrated that the combination of **pembrolizumab** (anti-PD-1) and **axitinib** (VEGF inhibitor) significantly improved **overall survival** and **response rates** compared to sunitinib alone, leading to FDA approval of the combination for first-line treatment in mRCC.

Adjuvant Therapy

In patients with **high-risk localized RCC** following nephrectomy, **adjuvant therapy** is a consideration to reduce the risk of recurrence.

- **Sunitinib**: The **S-TRAC trial** showed that adjuvant **sunitinib** improved **disease-free survival** compared to placebo in patients with high-risk RCC, leading to its approval for adjuvant use. However, its benefit in terms of overall survival has been debated, and adjuvant therapy remains an individualized decision based on patient risk factors and preferences.

6.10.3. Latest Advances in Kidney Cancer Treatment

Significant advances have been made in the treatment of **advanced and metastatic kidney cancer**, particularly with the integration of **immunotherapy** and **combination therapies**.

Immune Checkpoint Inhibitors (ICIs)

Immune checkpoint inhibitors have revolutionized the treatment of RCC, particularly in advanced disease.

- **Nivolumab and Ipilimumab**: As previously mentioned, the **CheckMate 214 trial** established the combination of **nivolumab** (anti-PD-1) and **ipilimumab** (anti-CTLA-4) as a superior treatment for patients with intermediate- and poor-risk mRCC. The trial demonstrated improved **overall survival** and **response rates**, with a durable response in many patients, making it a preferred first-line therapy.
- **Pembrolizumab and Axitinib**: The combination of **pembrolizumab** and **axitinib** has also shown impressive results in **KEYNOTE-426**, where patients receiving the combination had a 47% reduction in the risk of death compared to those receiving sunitinib alone. This combination has become a new standard for first-line treatment in mRCC.

Targeted Therapies

Tyrosine kinase inhibitors (TKIs) continue to play a central role in the treatment of RCC, particularly for patients who cannot receive immunotherapy or who have progressed on ICIs.

- **Cabozantinib**: **Cabozantinib**, a multi-kinase inhibitor targeting VEGF, MET, and AXL, has shown improved survival in both the **first-line** and **second-line** settings. The **CABOSUN trial** demonstrated that cabozantinib improved **progression-free survival** compared to sunitinib in patients with intermediate- and poor-risk disease.
- **Lenvatinib and Everolimus**: The combination of **lenvatinib** (a TKI) and **everolimus** (an mTOR inhibitor) has shown efficacy in patients who have progressed on VEGF-targeted therapies. The **Study 205** trial demonstrated improved **progression-free survival** with the combination compared to everolimus alone in pretreated patients.

6.11. Liver Cancer (Hepatocellular Carcinoma)

Liver cancer, predominantly **hepatocellular carcinoma (HCC)**, is a major cause of cancer-related deaths worldwide, with a particularly high incidence in regions where chronic viral hepatitis is prevalent. The increasing burden of liver cancer, particularly due to the global rise in **nonalcoholic fatty liver disease (NAFLD)**, has led to significant advancements in screening, diagnosis, and treatment options.

6.11.1. Screening for Liver Cancer

Effective **screening** for liver cancer is crucial for improving outcomes, as early detection allows for curative treatments. Screening is recommended for **high-risk individuals** based on the presence of known risk factors such as chronic liver disease, viral hepatitis, or cirrhosis.

Screening Guidelines

The **NCCN guidelines** recommend **regular screening** for individuals at high risk of developing hepatocellular carcinoma (HCC). High-risk populations include:

- **Patients with cirrhosis**: Due to any cause, including **hepatitis B** or **hepatitis C, alcoholic liver disease**, or **nonalcoholic steatohepatitis (NASH)**.
- **Chronic hepatitis B infection**: Even without cirrhosis, chronic hepatitis B (especially in patients of Asian or African descent) is a significant risk factor for HCC, and these patients should be regularly screened.
- **Family history of HCC**: Individuals with a family history of liver cancer should also undergo routine surveillance.

Screening Modalities

The **NCCN guidelines** recommend screening with **ultrasound** every **6 months**, with or without the use of **serum alpha-fetoprotein (AFP)** levels, for at-risk populations.

- **Ultrasound**: The primary modality for screening due to its non-invasive nature and relative cost-effectiveness. Studies have shown that regular ultrasound screening improves early detection rates, which correlates with better survival outcomes.
- **Alpha-Fetoprotein (AFP)**: Serum **AFP** is often used in conjunction with ultrasound for surveillance. Elevated AFP levels can indicate the presence of HCC, but its utility as a sole screening tool is limited due to false positives and low sensitivity in early-stage disease. A study by **Marrero et al. (2009)** indicated that combining AFP with ultrasound increases the sensitivity of screening for HCC, but AFP alone is insufficient for early detection.

6.11.2. Risk Factors for Liver Cancer

The development of liver cancer is strongly associated with underlying **chronic liver disease** and specific **modifiable** and **non-modifiable risk factors**. Understanding these risk factors is essential for targeting prevention efforts and identifying individuals who would benefit most from screening.

Chronic Hepatitis B and C Infections

Chronic viral hepatitis is the most significant risk factor for HCC worldwide:

- **Hepatitis B Virus (HBV)**: Chronic infection with **hepatitis B** is a leading cause of HCC, particularly in **Asia** and **Africa**, where HBV is endemic. HBV promotes liver inflammation, fibrosis, and carcinogenesis. Studies have demonstrated that **antiviral therapy** for chronic hepatitis B can reduce the risk of HCC by controlling viral replication and preventing disease progression.
- **Hepatitis C Virus (HCV): Chronic hepatitis C infection** is a major risk factor for HCC, especially in the **United States** and **Europe. Direct-acting antiviral (DAA) therapy** for HCV has significantly reduced the incidence of HCC by curing the infection and

preventing liver disease progression. However, HCV-cured individuals with advanced fibrosis or cirrhosis remain at risk and require continued surveillance.

Alcohol and Nonalcoholic Fatty Liver Disease (NAFLD)

- **Alcoholic Liver Disease**: Chronic alcohol consumption leads to **cirrhosis**, significantly increasing the risk of HCC. Studies have demonstrated that long-term alcohol abuse is a direct contributor to liver carcinogenesis.
- **Nonalcoholic Fatty Liver Disease (NAFLD)/Nonalcoholic Steatohepatitis (NASH)**: NAFLD, particularly its progressive form, **NASH**, is becoming a leading cause of liver cancer in the **Western world**, driven by rising obesity and metabolic syndrome. Studies by **Younossi et al. (2019)** have shown that the incidence of HCC related to NASH has increased significantly, even in the absence of cirrhosis, making it an emerging concern for hepatologists.

Other Risk Factors

Other notable risk factors for liver cancer include:

- **Diabetes and Obesity**: **Diabetes mellitus** and **obesity** are independently associated with an increased risk of HCC, likely due to their contribution to **NAFLD** and **insulin resistance**, which promote liver inflammation and fibrosis.
- **Aflatoxin Exposure**: In certain regions, particularly **Sub-Saharan Africa** and **Asia**, exposure to **aflatoxins** (toxins produced by molds in improperly stored grains) is a known carcinogen that increases HCC risk.

6.11.3. Treatment of Liver Cancer: NCCN Guidelines

The treatment of liver cancer is highly dependent on the **stage of the disease** at diagnosis, the extent of liver function, and the patient's performance status. **NCCN guidelines** emphasize a **multidisciplinary approach** to HCC treatment, incorporating **surgery**, **ablation**, **embolization**, **systemic therapies**, and **liver transplantation**.

Curative Treatments for Early-Stage Disease

For patients diagnosed at an early stage (typically via surveillance), curative options include:

- **Surgical Resection**: Surgical resection is the treatment of choice for patients with **localized HCC** and preserved liver function. **NCCN guidelines** recommend partial hepatectomy for patients with **Child-Pugh class A** liver function and a single, resectable tumor. Studies have shown that patients who undergo resection for early-stage HCC can achieve **5-year survival rates** exceeding 60%.
- **Liver Transplantation**: **Liver transplantation** is the definitive treatment for patients with early-stage HCC who have underlying cirrhosis and are not candidates for resection. Patients who meet the **Milan criteria** (a single tumor ≤5 cm or up to three

tumors ≤3 cm each) have excellent outcomes with transplantation, with **5-year survival rates** approaching 70%. A study by **Mazzaferro et al. (1996)** demonstrated that transplantation within the Milan criteria offers similar survival to non-cancer patients undergoing liver transplants.
- **Ablation Therapies**: For patients who are not candidates for surgery or transplantation, **ablation therapies** (such as **radiofrequency ablation [RFA]** or **microwave ablation [MWA]**) are effective in destroying small tumors. **RFA** is considered curative for tumors <3 cm, with comparable outcomes to resection in select patients.

Intermediate and Locally Advanced Disease

For patients with **intermediate or locally advanced HCC**, **locoregional therapies** are the mainstay of treatment.

- **Transarterial Chemoembolization (TACE)**: TACE is a widely used treatment for patients with **intermediate-stage HCC** who are not candidates for surgery or transplantation. TACE involves the selective delivery of chemotherapy and embolic agents directly into the hepatic artery, cutting off blood supply to the tumor. Studies have shown that **TACE** improves survival in patients with preserved liver function, with the **BRIDGE study** reporting a **median survival** of over 26 months.
- **Radioembolization (TARE)**: **Transarterial radioembolization (TARE)** with **yttrium-90** microspheres is another locoregional therapy that delivers radioactive particles directly to the tumor. It is an option for patients with larger or multifocal tumors. **SARAH and SIRveNIB trials** showed that **TARE** was comparable to **sorafenib** (systemic therapy) in terms of survival, with fewer side effects.

Systemic Therapy for Advanced and Metastatic Disease

For patients with **advanced-stage HCC** (stage C, BCLC classification), **systemic therapies** are the mainstay of treatment.

- **Tyrosine Kinase Inhibitors (TKIs)**: **Sorafenib**, a multikinase inhibitor, has been the standard first-line treatment for advanced HCC for over a decade. The **SHARP trial** demonstrated that sorafenib significantly improved **overall survival** (10.7 months vs. 7.9 months with placebo). **Lenvatinib**, another TKI, was shown in the **REFLECT trial** to be non-inferior to sorafenib, offering another option for first-line treatment.
- **Immunotherapy**: The **IMbrave150 trial** marked a major advance with the combination of **atezolizumab (PD-L1 inhibitor)** and **bevacizumab (anti-VEGF)**, which demonstrated superior outcomes compared to sorafenib. Patients treated with this combination had a **median overall survival of 19.2 months** compared to 13.4 months with sorafenib. This has led to **atezolizumab/bevacizumab** being recommended as a preferred first-line treatment in the **NCCN guidelines** for advanced HCC.
- **Second-Line Therapies**: For patients who progress on first-line therapy, options include TKIs such as **regorafenib** and **cabozantinib**, as well as **immune checkpoint inhibitors** like **nivolumab** and **pembrolizumab**. Studies such as the **RESORCE trial**

showed that **regorafenib** significantly improved survival in patients who had progressed on sorafenib.

6.11.4. Latest Updates in Liver Cancer Treatment

The most significant recent advancements in HCC treatment have been the introduction of **combination immunotherapy** and **TKI therapies**, as well as a better understanding of locoregional therapy indications.

Immunotherapy Advances

The combination of **immune checkpoint inhibitors** (e.g., **atezolizumab**) with **anti-VEGF therapy** (e.g., **bevacizumab**) has shown superior efficacy compared to TKIs alone, leading to a shift in the first-line treatment of advanced HCC.

- The **IMbrave150 trial** demonstrated that this combination significantly improved **overall survival** and **progression-free survival** compared to sorafenib, marking a new standard of care for patients with advanced HCC.

Novel Targeted Therapies

Research continues into other **targeted therapies** and **combinations** for advanced HCC. Drugs targeting specific mutations (e.g., **FGFR inhibitors** for patients with FGFR mutations) are under investigation, and combination strategies involving TKIs and immunotherapy are expected to further improve outcomes.

6.12. Esophageal Cancer

Esophageal cancer is a highly aggressive malignancy with poor survival rates, primarily because most cases are diagnosed at an advanced stage. There are two main histological types: **adenocarcinoma** and **squamous cell carcinoma**, each with distinct risk factors and geographic prevalence. The treatment of esophageal cancer has evolved significantly with advances in surgery, chemotherapy, radiation, and immunotherapy.

6.12.1. Screening for Esophageal Cancer

Routine screening for esophageal cancer in the general population is **not recommended** due to the low overall incidence. However, certain high-risk groups, especially those with **Barrett's esophagus**, may benefit from surveillance to detect early changes that could lead to **adenocarcinoma**.

Screening Guidelines for High-Risk Populations

Screening and surveillance efforts are focused on patients with **Barrett's esophagus**, a premalignant condition in which the normal squamous lining of the esophagus is replaced by columnar epithelium due to chronic **gastroesophageal reflux disease (GERD)**.

- **Barrett's Esophagus Surveillance**: Patients diagnosed with Barrett's esophagus are typically screened with **upper endoscopy (esophagogastroduodenoscopy, EGD)** and **biopsies** to detect dysplasia or early signs of adenocarcinoma. According to **NCCN guidelines**, patients with **low-grade dysplasia** may be screened every **6-12 months**, while those with **high-grade dysplasia** should be offered **endoscopic eradication therapy** or more frequent surveillance.

Endoscopic Screening

Endoscopic screening with **EGD** is recommended for patients with **chronic GERD**, especially those with additional risk factors such as obesity, male gender, Caucasian ethnicity, or age over 50 years. Studies such as the **BOSS trial** have demonstrated that early detection of **Barrett's esophagus** and subsequent surveillance can reduce the incidence of esophageal adenocarcinoma by detecting and treating dysplasia before it progresses.

- **Non-Endoscopic Screening**: Novel approaches like **Cytosponge**, a minimally invasive device used to collect cells from the esophagus for biomarker analysis, are being investigated for early detection of Barrett's esophagus and esophageal cancer in high-risk individuals. Early studies suggest this method may be a more cost-effective and less invasive alternative to endoscopy.

6.12.2. Risk Factors for Esophageal Cancer

The risk factors for esophageal cancer differ between **adenocarcinoma** and **squamous cell carcinoma**. Understanding these factors helps guide prevention strategies and screening efforts.

Risk Factors for Esophageal Adenocarcinoma

Esophageal adenocarcinoma primarily arises from **Barrett's esophagus**, which is often a consequence of chronic GERD. Major risk factors include:

- **Gastroesophageal Reflux Disease (GERD)**: Chronic GERD increases the risk of Barrett's esophagus and, subsequently, adenocarcinoma. Patients with frequent acid reflux are at significantly higher risk.
- **Barrett's Esophagus**: **Barrett's esophagus** is the most well-established precursor to adenocarcinoma. The progression from **Barrett's** to adenocarcinoma involves a multistep process of metaplasia to dysplasia, and finally to invasive cancer.
- **Obesity**: **Obesity**, particularly central obesity, is a strong risk factor for esophageal adenocarcinoma. The **Nexø et al. (2016)** study demonstrated that obese individuals have a more than **twofold increased risk** of developing esophageal adenocarcinoma.
- **Smoking**: **Smoking** contributes to both adenocarcinoma and squamous cell carcinoma of the esophagus. A **meta-analysis** by **Abnet et al. (2018)** confirmed that smoking remains a significant modifiable risk factor for esophageal adenocarcinoma.

- **Diet**: A diet high in processed meats and low in fruits and vegetables may also increase the risk of adenocarcinoma. Additionally, low intake of antioxidants and certain micronutrients has been associated with a higher risk of Barrett's esophagus progressing to cancer

Risk Factors for Squamous Cell Carcinoma

Esophageal squamous cell carcinoma has distinct risk factors and is more common in **Asia** and **Eastern Europe**. Key risk factors include:

- **Tobacco and Alcohol Use**: The combination of **heavy smoking** and **alcohol consumption** is a major risk factor for squamous cell carcinoma. **Alcohol consumption**, particularly of spirits, has been shown to have a synergistic effect with tobacco in increasing cancer risk. A **case-control study** by **Castellsagué et al. (1999)** demonstrated that individuals who smoked heavily and consumed large amounts of alcohol had a **50-fold higher risk** of esophageal squamous cell carcinoma than non-smokers and non-drinkers.
- **Dietary Factors**: Diets low in fruits and vegetables are associated with a higher risk of squamous cell carcinoma. In some regions, the consumption of foods high in **nitrosamines**, such as **preserved meats**, is also linked to an increased risk.
- **Esophageal Injury**: Injury to the esophagus from substances like **lye**, hot beverages, or radiation can increase the risk of squamous cell carcinoma.

6.12.3. Treatment of Esophageal Cancer: NCCN Guidelines

The **NCCN guidelines** for esophageal cancer emphasize a **multidisciplinary approach** that includes **surgery**, **chemoradiation**, **systemic therapy**, and **endoscopic therapies** depending on the stage of the disease. Treatment is typically stratified based on **resectability** and the patient's **performance status**.

Early-Stage Esophageal Cancer

For patients with **early-stage (T1, T2)** esophageal cancer, particularly those with **high-grade dysplasia** or **superficial tumors**, treatment focuses on **endoscopic resection** or surgery.

- **Endoscopic Mucosal Resection (EMR)**: For patients with **high-grade dysplasia** or **early T1 tumors**, EMR or **endoscopic submucosal dissection (ESD)** can be curative. Studies have shown that these endoscopic techniques are highly effective in eradicating early-stage tumors with low morbidity compared to esophagectomy.
- **Esophagectomy**: For patients with **T2 tumors** or tumors that have invaded deeper layers of the esophageal wall, **esophagectomy** is the treatment of choice. **Minimally invasive esophagectomy (MIE)** has shown to have comparable survival outcomes with open esophagectomy but with reduced complications. The **MIE Trial (2015)** demonstrated better short-term outcomes and faster recovery with the minimally invasive approach compared to traditional open surgery.

Locally Advanced Esophageal Cancer

For patients with **locally advanced esophageal cancer (T3, T4, N+)**, a **multimodal approach** is typically recommended, including **chemoradiation** followed by surgery or definitive chemoradiation in unresectable cases.

- **Neoadjuvant Chemoradiation**: **NCCN guidelines** recommend **neoadjuvant chemoradiation** for resectable **locally advanced** disease, based on the **CROSS trial**. The **CROSS trial** demonstrated that patients with **stage II/III esophageal cancer** treated with **neoadjuvant chemoradiation (carboplatin/paclitaxel + radiation)** followed by surgery had a significantly improved **overall survival (OS)** compared to surgery alone. The **5-year survival rate** for patients who received chemoradiation was **47%** compared to **34%** for those who had surgery alone.
- **Definitive Chemoradiation**: For patients who are not surgical candidates, **definitive chemoradiation** is an option. This treatment involves the combination of **radiotherapy** and **concurrent chemotherapy** to achieve local control.

Metastatic Esophageal Cancer

For patients with **metastatic disease (stage IV)**, treatment is palliative and focuses on prolonging survival and improving quality of life through **systemic therapy**.

- **Systemic Chemotherapy**: **Cisplatin** and **5-fluorouracil (5-FU)** are the traditional chemotherapy agents used in esophageal cancer. For adenocarcinoma, **FOLFOX (5-FU, leucovorin, oxaliplatin)** is a widely used regimen. Combination chemotherapy can improve response rates, but the prognosis remains poor.
- **Immunotherapy**: Recent advances have led to the incorporation of **immune checkpoint inhibitors** in the treatment of advanced esophageal cancer. The **KEYNOTE-181 trial** demonstrated that **pembrolizumab** (a PD-1 inhibitor) significantly improved survival in patients with **PD-L1-positive metastatic esophageal cancer**, particularly those with squamous cell carcinoma. Based on these findings, **NCCN guidelines** now recommend pembrolizumab for second-line treatment of PD-L1-positive esophageal cancer.

6.12.4. Latest Advances in Esophageal Cancer Treatment

Significant advances in the treatment of esophageal cancer have occurred, particularly with the use of **immunotherapy** and new **targeted therapies**.

Immunotherapy

The integration of **immune checkpoint inhibitors** has transformed the management of advanced esophageal cancer.

- **Pembrolizumab**: The **KEYNOTE-590 trial** demonstrated that **pembrolizumab**, in combination with chemotherapy, improved overall survival and progression-free survival

in patients with locally advanced or metastatic esophageal cancer, regardless of histology. This led to the FDA approval of pembrolizumab in combination with chemotherapy for the first-line treatment of advanced esophageal cancer.
- **Nivolumab**: The **CheckMate 648 trial** explored the role of **nivolumab** in combination with chemotherapy for squamous cell carcinoma of the esophagus. Results showed improved overall survival compared to chemotherapy alone, leading to FDA approval of **nivolumab** as a first-line treatment for advanced squamous cell carcinoma.

Targeted Therapies

- **Trastuzumab**: For patients with **HER2-positive esophageal adenocarcinoma**, **trastuzumab** has shown improved outcomes when added to chemotherapy. The **ToGA trial** demonstrated that adding trastuzumab to **cisplatin/5-FU** improved overall survival in patients with HER2-positive tumors.

6.13. Gastric Cancer

Gastric cancer, or stomach cancer, remains one of the leading causes of cancer-related mortality worldwide, especially in East Asia. Its incidence varies geographically, and despite declining rates in many regions, outcomes remain poor due to late-stage diagnosis. The introduction of **targeted therapies** and **immunotherapy** in recent years has improved the treatment landscape for advanced cases.

6.13.1. Screening for Gastric Cancer

Routine screening for gastric cancer is not common in many countries, but in high-incidence regions like **East Asia** (Japan, South Korea, China), screening is recommended due to the high prevalence of the disease and improved outcomes from early detection.

Screening Guidelines in High-Risk Populations

Screening efforts for gastric cancer are focused on populations at **high risk**, especially in countries where the incidence of gastric cancer is high. The **NCCN guidelines** recommend screening for patients with specific high-risk factors, particularly those with a family history of gastric cancer or certain genetic conditions.

- **Endoscopy**: In **Japan** and **South Korea**, **upper endoscopy** (esophagogastroduodenoscopy, or EGD) is widely used for gastric cancer screening, typically starting at age **40-50**. Regular endoscopic screening in these countries has been associated with the detection of early-stage cancers and improved survival rates.
- **Helicobacter pylori (H. pylori) Testing**: **H. pylori infection** is a significant risk factor for gastric cancer. In high-risk populations, **H. pylori testing and eradication** may reduce the risk of gastric cancer. The **NCCN guidelines** suggest that patients with chronic H. pylori infection who are at increased risk for gastric cancer should undergo eradication therapy, particularly in regions with high gastric cancer incidence.

Screening in Familial Syndromes

For individuals with **hereditary syndromes** that increase the risk of gastric cancer, such as **hereditary diffuse gastric cancer (HDGC)** associated with **CDH1 mutations**, the **NCCN guidelines** recommend regular screening with endoscopy or, in some cases, **prophylactic gastrectomy**.

- **Prophylactic Gastrectomy**: Patients with confirmed **CDH1 mutations** are at very high risk for **diffuse gastric cancer**, and prophylactic removal of the stomach may be recommended, even if no cancer has been detected, to prevent the development of aggressive cancers.

6.13.2. Risk Factors for Gastric Cancer

Understanding the risk factors for gastric cancer is essential for prevention and early detection. The most significant risk factors include **H. pylori infection**, **dietary factors**, and certain **genetic conditions**.

Helicobacter pylori Infection

H. pylori infection is the most significant risk factor for gastric cancer, particularly for **non-cardia gastric cancer** (cancer occurring in the lower part of the stomach). Chronic **H. pylori** infection induces inflammation of the gastric lining, leading to **atrophic gastritis**, **intestinal metaplasia**, and eventually cancer.

- **Eradication of H. pylori**: Studies have shown that **H. pylori eradication** can reduce the incidence of gastric cancer, particularly when eradication occurs before precancerous lesions develop. In a meta-analysis by **Ford et al. (2014)**, H. pylori eradication was associated with a **34% reduction** in the risk of developing gastric cancer in infected individuals.

Diet and Lifestyle

Dietary and lifestyle factors significantly contribute to the development of gastric cancer, particularly in Western countries.

- **Diet**: Diets high in **salt, processed meats, smoked foods**, and **pickled vegetables** are associated with an increased risk of gastric cancer. Conversely, a diet rich in **fresh fruits** and **vegetables** may reduce the risk.
- **Smoking and Alcohol**: **Smoking** is a known risk factor for gastric cancer, particularly for cancers of the upper stomach (cardia). **Alcohol consumption**, especially heavy use, also increases the risk of gastric cancer, particularly in conjunction with smoking.

Genetic Factors

Certain genetic syndromes increase the risk of gastric cancer.

- **Hereditary Diffuse Gastric Cancer (HDGC)**: This is an autosomal dominant condition associated with **CDH1 mutations**, significantly increasing the risk of **diffuse gastric cancer**. These individuals are often advised to undergo **prophylactic gastrectomy** due to the high lifetime risk of cancer development.
- **Familial Adenomatous Polyposis (FAP)** and **Lynch Syndrome**: Both syndromes are associated with an increased risk of gastric cancer, particularly in populations where gastric cancer screening is less common.

6.13.3. Treatment of Gastric Cancer: NCCN Guidelines

The **NCCN guidelines** for gastric cancer emphasize a multidisciplinary approach, with treatment strategies depending on the **stage of the disease**, **tumor location**, and **patient performance status**. Treatment involves a combination of **surgery, chemotherapy, radiation**, and, more recently, **immunotherapy** and **targeted therapies**.

Early-Stage Disease (Stage I)

For patients with **early-stage gastric cancer**, particularly **T1N0 tumors**, surgery is the primary treatment.

- **Endoscopic Mucosal Resection (EMR) or Endoscopic Submucosal Dissection (ESD)**: In patients with **very early-stage disease (T1a)**, **endoscopic resection** can be curative. Studies have shown that EMR or ESD achieves excellent outcomes with less morbidity than traditional surgery for early gastric cancers confined to the mucosa.
- **Subtotal or Total Gastrectomy**: For patients with more advanced early-stage disease (T1b or T2), **subtotal gastrectomy** (for distal tumors) or **total gastrectomy** (for proximal tumors) with lymph node dissection is recommended.

Locally Advanced Disease (Stages II and III)

For patients with **locally advanced disease**, a **multimodal approach** involving **surgery, chemotherapy**, and **radiation therapy** is the standard of care.

- **Neoadjuvant Chemotherapy**: The **NCCN guidelines** recommend **neoadjuvant chemotherapy** for patients with stage **II-III gastric cancer** before surgery. The **MAGIC trial** demonstrated that patients treated with **perioperative chemotherapy (epirubicin, cisplatin, and 5-FU)** had improved **overall survival (OS)** compared to those treated with surgery alone. **FLOT (5-fluorouracil, leucovorin, oxaliplatin, docetaxel)** is now also considered a preferred regimen based on the **FLOT4 trial**, which showed improved outcomes compared to the older MAGIC regimen.
- **Surgery**: Surgery is the mainstay of treatment for patients with locally advanced disease. **Radical gastrectomy with D2 lymphadenectomy** (removal of regional lymph nodes) is the standard procedure, offering the best chance for cure.
- **Adjuvant Chemotherapy or Chemoradiation**: For patients with positive margins or lymph node involvement following surgery, **adjuvant chemoradiation** (radiation

combined with chemotherapy) is recommended. The **INT-0116 trial** demonstrated that postoperative chemoradiation improves **disease-free survival (DFS)** and **overall survival** compared to surgery alone.

Metastatic or Advanced Disease (Stage IV)

For patients with **metastatic gastric cancer**, treatment is primarily palliative, aiming to prolong survival and relieve symptoms.

- **Systemic Chemotherapy**: **Cisplatin-based chemotherapy** (combined with fluoropyrimidines such as 5-FU or capecitabine) has been the backbone of treatment for advanced gastric cancer. The **ToGA trial** demonstrated that adding **trastuzumab**, a monoclonal antibody targeting **HER2**, to chemotherapy significantly improved **overall survival** in patients with **HER2-positive gastric cancer**.
- **Targeted Therapies**: In addition to **trastuzumab** for HER2-positive tumors, **ramucirumab**, a **VEGF receptor 2 (VEGFR2) inhibitor**, is approved as second-line therapy in combination with paclitaxel for advanced gastric cancer. The **RAINBOW trial** showed that **ramucirumab** improved overall survival in patients with previously treated metastatic gastric cancer.
- **Immunotherapy**: **Immunotherapy** has emerged as a promising treatment for advanced gastric cancer. The **KEYNOTE-061 trial** showed that **pembrolizumab**, an anti-PD-1 monoclonal antibody, improved outcomes in patients with **PD-L1-positive** gastric cancer. Pembrolizumab is now recommended as a second-line treatment in **NCCN guidelines** for patients with PD-L1-positive tumors.

6.13.4. Latest Advances in Gastric Cancer Treatment

Significant advancements have been made in the treatment of advanced gastric cancer, particularly with **immunotherapy** and **targeted therapies**.

Immunotherapy

Immunotherapy has gained prominence in the treatment of **advanced gastric cancer**, particularly for patients whose tumors express **PD-L1**.

- **Pembrolizumab**: The **KEYNOTE-590 trial** showed that pembrolizumab, when used in combination with chemotherapy, significantly improved **overall survival** in patients with advanced **PD-L1-positive gastric cancer**. This led to its FDA approval as a first-line treatment in combination with chemotherapy for patients with **PD-L1-positive tumors**.

Targeted Therapies

- **Trastuzumab Deruxtecan**: For patients with **HER2-positive gastric cancer** who have progressed on trastuzumab, **trastuzumab deruxtecan** has shown promising results. The **DESTINY-Gastric01 trial** demonstrated that trastuzumab deruxtecan improved

response rates and **overall survival** compared to chemotherapy in patients with HER2-positive advanced gastric cancer.
- **Ramucirumab**: As mentioned, **ramucirumab** is used in combination with **paclitaxel** for second-line treatment in patients with advanced gastric cancer. Its role continues to expand as trials explore its efficacy in combination with other agents.

Liquid Biopsies and Molecular Profiling

The use of **liquid biopsies** to detect circulating tumor DNA (ctDNA) and other biomarkers is being explored to guide treatment decisions and monitor disease progression. Molecular profiling of tumors to identify actionable mutations is becoming increasingly important in tailoring therapies to individual patients.

6.14. Melanoma

Melanoma, a highly aggressive form of skin cancer, arises from the malignant transformation of melanocytes, the cells responsible for producing pigment in the skin. Though it accounts for only 1% of all skin cancers, it causes the majority of skin cancer-related deaths due to its tendency to metastasize. Early detection and advancements in **targeted therapies** and **immunotherapies** have significantly improved outcomes.

6.14.1. Screening for Melanoma

Screening for melanoma focuses on the early detection of suspicious skin lesions, as early-stage melanoma is highly curable. Routine population-wide screening is not generally recommended, but **self-examinations, dermatologic assessments**, and the use of **dermoscopy** are important tools for detecting melanoma early in **high-risk individuals**.

Visual Skin Examinations

Skin self-examinations and **clinical skin examinations** by healthcare providers are the main methods of screening for melanoma. Patients are encouraged to monitor changes in their skin, particularly those related to **moles** or **pigmented lesions**, using the **ABCDE criteria** (Asymmetry, Border irregularity, Color variation, Diameter >6mm, Evolving).

- **Dermatologist-Performed Examinations**: High-risk individuals, such as those with a personal or family history of melanoma, should have **regular full-body skin exams** by a dermatologist. **NCCN guidelines** recommend these individuals undergo **clinical skin exams** every **6 to 12 months** depending on their risk profile.

Dermoscopy

Dermoscopy is a non-invasive diagnostic tool that enhances the visualization of skin lesions and helps differentiate benign from malignant lesions. Studies, such as those by **Kittler et al. (2002)**, have shown that dermoscopy improves the diagnostic accuracy of melanoma detection, leading to earlier treatment and better outcomes.

Total Body Photography and Digital Monitoring

In patients with multiple moles or atypical nevi, **total body photography** or **digital mole mapping** can be helpful in monitoring for changes over time. **Sequential digital dermoscopic imaging** (SDDI) has been shown to detect melanomas that may not meet typical clinical criteria, particularly in high-risk patients.

Screening Guidelines in High-Risk Populations

While population-wide screening for melanoma is not recommended, **NCCN guidelines** suggest that high-risk individuals, such as those with **atypical mole syndrome**, **immunosuppression**, or a **family history of melanoma**, should undergo regular dermatologic evaluations. These patients may also benefit from **genetic counseling** and testing for mutations in **CDKN2A** and other genes associated with familial melanoma syndromes.

6.14.2. Risk Factors for Melanoma

There are several well-established **risk factors** for developing melanoma, including **genetic predispositions, UV radiation exposure**, and **phenotypic characteristics**.

UV Radiation Exposure

Ultraviolet (UV) radiation exposure from the sun and artificial sources (such as tanning beds) is the most significant environmental risk factor for melanoma.

- **Intermittent Sun Exposure**: Melanoma is more strongly associated with **intermittent intense sun exposure**, particularly in childhood, rather than chronic exposure. **Whiteman et al. (2001)** showed that patients with a history of blistering sunburns during childhood or adolescence had a **twofold increased risk** of developing melanoma.
- **Tanning Beds**: The use of **indoor tanning devices** significantly increases the risk of melanoma. A large meta-analysis by **Colantonio et al. (2014)** found that individuals who used tanning beds had a **20% increased risk** of melanoma, with the risk being even higher for those who began using tanning beds before age 35.

Genetic Factors

Several **genetic mutations** and familial syndromes increase the risk of developing melanoma:

- **CDKN2A Mutation**: Mutations in the **CDKN2A gene** are linked to **familial melanoma syndromes**, which account for approximately **5-10% of melanoma cases**. These individuals often develop melanoma at a younger age and may have multiple primary tumors.
- **MC1R Gene**: Variants in the **MC1R gene**, which affect pigmentation, are also associated with an increased risk of melanoma, particularly in individuals with **fair skin, red hair**, and **freckles**.

Phenotypic Characteristics

Certain phenotypic traits are associated with a higher risk of melanoma:

- **Fair Skin**: Individuals with **light skin**, **blue or green eyes**, and **red or blond hair** are at higher risk, particularly if they burn easily and have difficulty tanning.
- **Numerous Nevi**: Having a large number of moles (**>50 nevi**) or atypical moles significantly increases the risk of developing melanoma. Patients with **atypical mole syndrome** require regular surveillance.

Family History

A **family history of melanoma** increases the risk of developing the disease. Studies have shown that individuals with **first-degree relatives** affected by melanoma have a **2-3 fold higher risk** of developing melanoma themselves.

6.14.3. Treatment of Melanoma: NCCN Guidelines

Treatment for melanoma is based on the **stage** of the disease at diagnosis. The **NCCN guidelines** recommend a **multidisciplinary approach**, with surgery as the primary treatment for early-stage disease and **systemic therapies** (e.g., immunotherapy, targeted therapy) for advanced stages.

Early-Stage Melanoma (Stage I-II)

For **localized melanoma**, surgical excision is the mainstay of treatment. Early detection leads to high cure rates, as **stage I-II melanomas** have not yet metastasized.

- **Wide Local Excision (WLE)**: The primary treatment for **stage I-II melanoma** is **wide local excision** with appropriate margins, based on the **Breslow depth** of the tumor. For tumors <1 mm in thickness, **1 cm margins** are recommended, while thicker tumors require **2 cm margins**.
- **Sentinel Lymph Node Biopsy (SLNB)**: **Sentinel lymph node biopsy** is recommended for melanomas with a Breslow depth >1 mm or with other high-risk features (e.g., ulceration, high mitotic rate). Studies, such as the **MSLT-1 trial**, demonstrated that SLNB improves **staging accuracy** and provides prognostic information without improving overall survival. Patients with positive sentinel nodes may require a complete lymph node dissection.

Locally Advanced Melanoma (Stage III)

For patients with **locoregionally advanced melanoma** (involvement of regional lymph nodes or in-transit metastases), treatment includes **surgery, adjuvant therapies**, and **immunotherapy**.

- **Surgical Lymphadenectomy**: For patients with nodal metastasis, **complete lymph node dissection** was previously standard. However, recent evidence, including the

MSLT-2 trial, demonstrated that patients with microscopic sentinel node involvement do not benefit from complete lymphadenectomy, leading to a more selective use of this procedure.

- **Adjuvant Therapy**: For patients with high-risk, resected melanoma, **adjuvant therapy** is recommended. **NCCN guidelines** now include **PD-1 inhibitors** (e.g., **nivolumab** or **pembrolizumab**) or **BRAF/MEK inhibitors** (e.g., **dabrafenib** and **trametinib**) for patients with **BRAF V600 mutations** as adjuvant therapy. The **CheckMate 238 trial** demonstrated that adjuvant nivolumab significantly improved **relapse-free survival (RFS)** compared to ipilimumab in patients with resected stage III and IV melanoma.

Metastatic or Unresectable Melanoma (Stage IV)

For patients with **metastatic melanoma** (stage IV) or unresectable disease, **systemic therapy** is the cornerstone of treatment. Advances in **immunotherapy** and **targeted therapies** have dramatically improved outcomes.

- **Checkpoint Inhibitors (Immunotherapy)**: Immune checkpoint inhibitors, particularly **PD-1 inhibitors** like **pembrolizumab** and **nivolumab**, have revolutionized the treatment of metastatic melanoma. The **KEYNOTE-006 trial** demonstrated that **pembrolizumab** significantly improved **overall survival (OS)** compared to ipilimumab in patients with advanced melanoma, leading to the widespread adoption of PD-1 inhibitors as first-line therapy.
- **BRAF/MEK Inhibitors**: For patients with **BRAF V600E/K mutations**, which occur in approximately **50% of melanomas**, BRAF inhibitors (e.g., **vemurafenib, dabrafenib**) combined with **MEK inhibitors** (e.g., **trametinib, cobimetinib**) are highly effective. The **COMBI-d trial** showed that the combination of **dabrafenib and trametinib** improved **progression-free survival (PFS)** and **overall survival** compared to monotherapy with dabrafenib.

Palliative Treatment for Advanced Melanoma

For patients with advanced melanoma that is not responsive to immunotherapy or targeted therapies, treatment focuses on palliation.

- **Radiation Therapy**: **Radiation therapy** can be used for palliation in patients with **brain metastases** or **painful bone metastases**. Stereotactic radiosurgery (SRS) is frequently used for melanoma brain metastases.

6.14.4. Latest Advances in Melanoma Treatment

Recent advances in the treatment of melanoma have focused on **immunotherapy**, **combination therapies**, and the exploration of **personalized medicine** based on genetic and molecular profiling.

Combination Immunotherapy

The combination of **nivolumab (PD-1 inhibitor)** and **ipilimumab (CTLA-4 inhibitor)** has been shown to produce durable responses in patients with advanced melanoma.

- The **CheckMate 067 trial** demonstrated that the combination of **nivolumab** and **ipilimumab** resulted in **5-year overall survival rates** of 52% in patients with metastatic melanoma, compared to 44% with nivolumab alone and 26% with ipilimumab alone. Combination therapy is now considered a standard option for first-line treatment of advanced melanoma in patients with good performance status.

Neo-Adjuvant Immunotherapy

Neo-adjuvant immunotherapy (immunotherapy given before surgery) is an area of active research. Early studies suggest that giving **PD-1 inhibitors** or **BRAF/MEK inhibitors** in the neo-adjuvant setting may reduce tumor burden and improve surgical outcomes for patients with resectable stage III melanoma.

Targeted Therapies for BRAF-Negative Melanomas

Researchers are exploring targeted therapies for melanomas without **BRAF mutations**, such as **NRAS-mutated** or **KIT-mutated** melanomas. **Selumetinib**, a MEK inhibitor, is being investigated for **NRAS-mutant melanoma**, though its efficacy is still under study.

6.15. Non-Hodgkin Lymphoma

Non-Hodgkin lymphoma (NHL) is a diverse group of blood cancers that develop from **lymphocytes**, a type of white blood cell involved in the immune system. NHL is classified into more than 60 subtypes, with **diffuse large B-cell lymphoma (DLBCL)** and **follicular lymphoma (FL)** being the most common. The disease can range from **indolent (slow-growing)** to **aggressive (fast-growing)** forms. Advances in **targeted therapy** and **immunotherapy** have revolutionized the treatment of NHL, significantly improving survival rates.

6.15.1. Screening for Non-Hodgkin Lymphoma

Routine population-based **screening** for NHL is not currently recommended because the incidence of the disease is relatively low, and no effective screening tests have been identified. NHL is typically diagnosed after the appearance of symptoms, which may include **painless lymphadenopathy**, **fever**, **night sweats**, **unexplained weight loss**, and **fatigue**.

High-Risk Populations

Screening efforts may be more appropriate for individuals at higher risk of developing NHL, such as those with underlying immunodeficiency, viral infections, or autoimmune diseases.

- **Immunosuppressed Patients**: Patients with **HIV/AIDS** or those undergoing chronic **immunosuppressive therapy** (e.g., for organ transplantation or autoimmune disease)

have an increased risk of developing NHL. For these individuals, close monitoring for early symptoms of NHL is critical.
- **Genetic Predisposition**: Individuals with genetic conditions such as **ataxia-telangiectasia** or **Wiskott-Aldrich syndrome** are also at increased risk and may benefit from closer medical surveillance, though no formal screening guidelines exist.

Blood Tests and Biomarkers

While there are no definitive screening tests for NHL, blood tests such as **complete blood counts (CBC)** and measurements of **lactate dehydrogenase (LDH)** can provide clues in high-risk patients. Elevated LDH is often seen in more aggressive subtypes of NHL and can be an early indicator of disease progression.

6.15.2. Risk Factors for Non-Hodgkin Lymphoma

Several **risk factors** have been identified that increase the likelihood of developing NHL. These risk factors can be **environmental**, **genetic**, or related to underlying health conditions.

Age and Gender

The incidence of NHL increases with **age**, and it is more common in **men** than in women. The median age of diagnosis is around **67 years**.

Immunosuppression

Chronic immunosuppression is a major risk factor for NHL:

- **HIV/AIDS**: People with **HIV** have a significantly higher risk of developing **aggressive B-cell lymphomas**, such as **primary CNS lymphoma** and **Burkitt lymphoma**. Studies have shown that antiretroviral therapy (ART) can reduce the incidence of NHL in HIV-infected individuals by restoring immune function.
- **Organ Transplant Recipients**: Recipients of **solid organ transplants** who require long-term immunosuppressive therapy (e.g., tacrolimus, cyclosporine) are at increased risk of NHL, particularly **post-transplant lymphoproliferative disorder (PTLD)**.

Infections

Several viral infections are associated with an increased risk of NHL:

- **Epstein-Barr Virus (EBV)**: EBV is strongly linked to **Burkitt lymphoma** and other NHL subtypes, particularly in immunocompromised patients. Studies suggest that **EBV-driven** lymphoproliferative disorders arise from the virus's ability to infect and transform B cells.
- **Hepatitis C Virus (HCV)**: Chronic **HCV infection** is associated with an increased risk of **marginal zone lymphoma** and **diffuse large B-cell lymphoma (DLBCL)**. **NHL cases**

related to HCV have been shown to respond to antiviral therapy, suggesting that viral eradication may reduce the risk of lymphoma development.

Autoimmune Diseases

Individuals with autoimmune diseases, such as **rheumatoid arthritis** and **Sjogren's syndrome**, have a higher risk of developing **marginal zone lymphoma** and other NHL subtypes. The chronic immune activation seen in these diseases may contribute to malignant transformation in lymphocytes.

Environmental and Occupational Exposures

Exposure to certain chemicals, including **pesticides** and **herbicides**, is associated with a higher risk of developing NHL. Studies have found an increased incidence of NHL in agricultural workers exposed to chemicals like **glyphosate**.

6.15.3. Treatment of Non-Hodgkin Lymphoma: NCCN Guidelines

Treatment for NHL is based on several factors, including the **specific subtype**, **stage of disease**, **patient performance status**, and **prognostic markers**. The **NCCN guidelines** for NHL emphasize **tailored treatment approaches** for the various subtypes, ranging from **watchful waiting** for indolent lymphomas to aggressive **chemotherapy** and **immunotherapy** for high-grade lymphomas.

Indolent Lymphomas (e.g., Follicular Lymphoma)

Indolent NHL, such as **follicular lymphoma**, tends to grow slowly and may not require immediate treatment upon diagnosis.

- **Watchful Waiting**: For asymptomatic patients with low tumor burden, **observation** is often recommended. Studies have shown that early intervention in asymptomatic indolent lymphomas does not improve overall survival, making **watchful waiting** a standard initial approach.
- **Rituximab (Monoclonal Antibody Therapy)**: For symptomatic or progressive disease, treatment usually involves **rituximab**, an anti-CD20 monoclonal antibody. The **PRIMA study** demonstrated that maintenance therapy with rituximab after initial treatment significantly improves **progression-free survival (PFS)** in follicular lymphoma patients.
- **Bendamustine and Rituximab (BR)**: For patients who require systemic therapy, the combination of **bendamustine and rituximab** is a commonly used regimen. The **STiL NHL1** trial found that BR had better progression-free survival rates and fewer side effects compared to R-CHOP (rituximab, cyclophosphamide, doxorubicin, vincristine, prednisone) in indolent NHL.

Aggressive Lymphomas (e.g., Diffuse Large B-Cell Lymphoma)

Diffuse large B-cell lymphoma (DLBCL) is the most common subtype of NHL and is classified as an **aggressive lymphoma**.

- **R-CHOP**: The standard treatment for **DLBCL** is **R-CHOP** (rituximab, cyclophosphamide, doxorubicin, vincristine, and prednisone). This regimen has been shown to result in long-term remissions in a significant proportion of patients with DLBCL. The landmark study by **Coiffier et al. (2002)** demonstrated that adding **rituximab** to CHOP significantly improved **overall survival** and **event-free survival** in elderly patients with DLBCL.
- **Radiation Therapy**: For patients with **early-stage (localized) DLBCL**, radiation therapy may be added to R-CHOP, particularly in cases where the disease is confined to a single site.
- **CNS Prophylaxis**: In patients with **high-risk features** (e.g., **high LDH levels**, involvement of **testes** or **sinuses**), **CNS prophylaxis** using intrathecal methotrexate is recommended to prevent central nervous system relapse.

Relapsed or Refractory Disease

For patients with **relapsed or refractory NHL**, several new treatment options have emerged:

- **CAR-T Cell Therapy**: **Chimeric antigen receptor (CAR) T-cell therapy**, such as **axicabtagene ciloleucel** and **tisagenlecleucel**, has shown remarkable efficacy in patients with **relapsed or refractory DLBCL**. The **ZUMA-1 trial** demonstrated durable remissions in heavily pretreated patients with DLBCL who received **CAR-T therapy**, leading to its FDA approval.
- **Polatuzumab Vedotin**: This antibody-drug conjugate targeting **CD79b** has been approved for patients with relapsed/refractory DLBCL when combined with **bendamustine** and **rituximab**. The **GO29365 trial** showed improved overall survival with this combination compared to bendamustine and rituximab alone.

Treatment of Other Subtypes

Different subtypes of NHL require tailored approaches:

- **Mantle Cell Lymphoma (MCL)**: The combination of **rituximab, bendamustine**, and **cytarabine** followed by **autologous stem cell transplantation** (ASCT) is considered standard for younger, fit patients with **mantle cell lymphoma**. **Ibrutinib**, a **BTK inhibitor**, has also shown efficacy in relapsed MCL.
- **Burkitt Lymphoma**: This highly aggressive lymphoma requires intensive **chemotherapy regimens** such as **CODOX-M/IVAC** (cyclophosphamide, doxorubicin, vincristine, methotrexate/ifosfamide, etoposide, cytarabine) to achieve long-term remission.

6.15.4. Latest Advances in NHL Treatment

The treatment of NHL has evolved significantly in recent years with the introduction of **targeted therapies, immunotherapy,** and **CAR-T cell therapy.**

CAR-T Cell Therapy

CAR-T cell therapy has revolutionized the treatment of **relapsed or refractory DLBCL** and **mantle cell lymphoma**.

- The **ZUMA-1 trial** showed that **axicabtagene ciloleucel** achieved **complete remissions** in over 50% of patients with refractory DLBCL, with some patients maintaining long-term remissions.

Bispecific Antibodies

Bispecific T-cell engagers (BiTEs), such as **blinatumomab**, are designed to bind both **T cells** and **B-cell antigens**, directing the immune system to target lymphoma cells.

- Early studies have shown that **blinatumomab** has activity in relapsed/refractory DLBCL and mantle cell lymphoma, and ongoing trials are evaluating its role in the frontline setting.

BTK Inhibitors

Bruton's tyrosine kinase (BTK) inhibitors, such as **ibrutinib**, have shown efficacy in several subtypes of NHL, particularly in **mantle cell lymphoma** and **chronic lymphocytic leukemia (CLL)**.

- The **RESONATE trial** demonstrated that **ibrutinib** significantly improved **progression-free survival** compared to **ofatumumab** in patients with relapsed or refractory CLL, leading to its approval for CLL and mantle cell lymphoma.

6.16. Hodgkin Lymphoma

Hodgkin lymphoma (HL) is a highly treatable form of lymphoma characterized by the presence of **Reed-Sternberg cells** in lymphatic tissue. It most commonly affects young adults but can also occur in older populations. Due to the development of highly effective treatment regimens, the prognosis for Hodgkin lymphoma has significantly improved, with high cure rates even for advanced stages.

6.16.1. Screening for Hodgkin Lymphoma

Routine screening for **Hodgkin lymphoma** in asymptomatic individuals is not recommended because it is a relatively rare disease and there are no effective screening tests for early detection. Hodgkin lymphoma is most commonly diagnosed when patients present with specific symptoms.

Clinical Presentation

Patients with Hodgkin lymphoma often present with the following **signs and symptoms**, which may warrant further investigation:

- **Painless lymphadenopathy**: Enlargement of lymph nodes, particularly in the **cervical** and **supraclavicular** regions, is the most common presenting sign. These lymph nodes are typically **non-tender** and may fluctuate in size.
- **B Symptoms**: Systemic symptoms, known as **B symptoms**, include **fever, night sweats**, and **unexplained weight loss**. These are often seen in more advanced cases and are associated with a poorer prognosis.
- **Fatigue** and **pruritus** are other common symptoms of Hodgkin lymphoma, though these are less specific.

Diagnosis

When Hodgkin lymphoma is suspected based on symptoms and physical examination, the diagnosis is confirmed through **biopsy** of an enlarged lymph node.

- **Excisional Biopsy**: A complete **lymph node excisional biopsy** is preferred to obtain enough tissue for histopathologic diagnosis, which includes identifying **Reed-Sternberg cells**.

6.16.2. Risk Factors for Hodgkin Lymphoma

Several **risk factors** have been identified for Hodgkin lymphoma, although the exact cause is not fully understood. The most notable risk factors include **viral infections, family history**, and **immune system dysregulation**.

Viral Infections

Epstein-Barr Virus (EBV) is the most significant viral risk factor for Hodgkin lymphoma. EBV is implicated in **30-50%** of cases, particularly in **mixed cellularity subtype** of HL.

- **Mechanism of EBV**: EBV infects B-cells, leading to their transformation and increased risk of malignant transformation. A study by **Hjalgrim et al. (2003)** demonstrated that individuals with **EBV-positive infectious mononucleosis** are at a higher risk of developing Hodgkin lymphoma.

Family History

A **family history of Hodgkin lymphoma** is a known risk factor. First-degree relatives of patients with Hodgkin lymphoma have a **3-5 fold increased risk** of developing the disease. Studies, such as those by **Kaldor et al. (1990)**, suggest that genetic susceptibility may play a role in disease development.

Immunosuppression

Individuals with compromised immune systems are at greater risk for developing Hodgkin lymphoma. This includes patients with:

- **HIV/AIDS**: Hodgkin lymphoma is more common in **HIV-positive individuals**, though the incidence has decreased with the advent of **antiretroviral therapy (ART)**.
- **Autoimmune Disorders**: Conditions such as **rheumatoid arthritis** and **systemic lupus erythematosus** have been associated with a higher incidence of HL, likely due to chronic immune activation and dysregulation.

Age and Gender

Hodgkin lymphoma has a **bimodal age distribution**, with a peak in incidence in **young adults** (ages 15-35) and another in **older adults** (over age 55). It is slightly more common in **men** than in women.

6.16.3. Treatment of Hodgkin Lymphoma: NCCN Guidelines

Treatment for Hodgkin lymphoma is highly effective, with **NCCN guidelines** outlining therapy based on the stage of the disease and the presence of **risk factors**. Treatment typically involves a combination of **chemotherapy**, **radiation**, and, in select cases, **immunotherapy** or **stem cell transplantation**.

Early-Stage Hodgkin Lymphoma (Stages I-II)

For patients with **early-stage (I-II) Hodgkin lymphoma**, treatment is based on the **favorable** or **unfavorable** risk profile of the disease.

- **Favorable Early-Stage HL**: These patients have no **B symptoms**, normal **ESR (erythrocyte sedimentation rate)**, and fewer than three involved lymph node regions. The NCCN guidelines recommend:
    - **ABVD Chemotherapy**: A standard chemotherapy regimen, consisting of **doxorubicin (Adriamycin), bleomycin, vinblastine**, and **dacarbazine** (ABVD), is typically given for 2-4 cycles.
    - **Involved-Site Radiation Therapy (ISRT)**: Radiation therapy is added after chemotherapy to reduce the risk of local recurrence, particularly in patients with bulky disease.
    - Studies, such as **Engert et al. (2010)**, have shown that combining **ABVD chemotherapy** with **radiation therapy** achieves cure rates exceeding **90%** in early-stage disease.
- **Unfavorable Early-Stage HL**: Patients with bulky disease, B symptoms, or elevated ESR may require more intensive treatment. The NCCN guidelines recommend:
    - **Escalated BEACOPP**: For patients with high-risk features, a more intensive regimen called **BEACOPP** (bleomycin, etoposide, doxorubicin,

cyclophosphamide, vincristine, procarbazine, prednisone) may be used to improve outcomes.

Advanced-Stage Hodgkin Lymphoma (Stages III-IV)

For **advanced-stage Hodgkin lymphoma**, treatment typically involves more cycles of chemotherapy, with or without radiation therapy.

- **ABVD or Escalated BEACOPP**: The NCCN guidelines recommend **ABVD** or **escalated BEACOPP** for patients with **advanced disease**. The **GHSG HD15 trial** demonstrated that escalated **BEACOPP** improved **progression-free survival** compared to ABVD in patients with advanced-stage disease, though at the cost of increased toxicity.
- **PET-Guided Therapy**: For advanced-stage disease, treatment is often guided by **interim PET-CT scans** performed after 2-4 cycles of chemotherapy. A **negative PET scan** may allow for de-escalation of therapy, reducing long-term toxicity. Studies like **Johnson et al. (2016)** showed that omitting **bleomycin** from later cycles in PET-negative patients reduces pulmonary toxicity without compromising outcomes.

Relapsed or Refractory Disease

For patients with **relapsed or refractory HL**, salvage therapy followed by **autologous stem cell transplantation (ASCT)** is the standard of care.

- **Salvage Chemotherapy**: ICE (ifosfamide, carboplatin, etoposide) or ESHAP (etoposide, methylprednisolone, cytarabine, cisplatin) are commonly used salvage regimens to induce remission before transplant.
- **Autologous Stem Cell Transplantation (ASCT)**: ASCT is recommended for patients who achieve remission with salvage chemotherapy. The **AETHERA trial** demonstrated that **brentuximab vedotin** (an anti-CD30 monoclonal antibody-drug conjugate) as maintenance therapy after ASCT significantly improves **progression-free survival** in high-risk patients.

Immunotherapy

For patients who are ineligible for ASCT or relapse after transplant, **immunotherapy** with **PD-1 inhibitors** has become an important treatment option.

- **Nivolumab and Pembrolizumab**: **Nivolumab** and **pembrolizumab** (PD-1 inhibitors) have shown remarkable activity in **relapsed/refractory Hodgkin lymphoma**. The **CheckMate 205 trial** demonstrated that nivolumab led to high response rates in heavily pretreated patients, with durable remissions in a significant subset of patients.

Treatment for Elderly Patients

For older adults with Hodgkin lymphoma, treatment must be adjusted to minimize toxicity while maintaining efficacy. **NCCN guidelines** suggest reduced-intensity regimens, such as **AAVD** (brentuximab vedotin, doxorubicin, vinblastine, dacarbazine), for older patients who cannot tolerate standard ABVD.

6.16.4. Latest Advances in Hodgkin Lymphoma Treatment

Several advances in the treatment of Hodgkin lymphoma have emerged in recent years, particularly the development of **immunotherapy** and **targeted therapies**.

Brentuximab Vedotin

Brentuximab vedotin is an **anti-CD30 antibody-drug conjugate** that has become a cornerstone of therapy for relapsed/refractory HL. It is now also being incorporated into frontline therapy for selected patients.

- The **ECHELON-1 trial** compared **AAVD (brentuximab vedotin, doxorubicin, vinblastine, dacarbazine)** with the standard **ABVD regimen**. The trial demonstrated improved **progression-free survival** for patients receiving AAVD, particularly those with stage III/IV disease. Brentuximab has since been FDA-approved as part of frontline therapy for advanced-stage Hodgkin lymphoma.

PD-1 Inhibitors

The introduction of **PD-1 inhibitors** (**nivolumab** and **pembrolizumab**) has changed the landscape for patients with **relapsed/refractory HL**.

- **Nivolumab and Pembrolizumab** are approved for the treatment of **relapsed HL** after failure of ASCT or brentuximab vedotin. Studies, such as the **KEYNOTE-087 trial**, demonstrated that **pembrolizumab** has durable activity in patients with relapsed/refractory HL, offering long-term remission for some patients.

Reduced-Intensity Chemotherapy

For older patients or those who cannot tolerate intensive therapy, **reduced-intensity regimens** incorporating **brentuximab** or **immunotherapy** are being explored to minimize toxicity while maintaining efficacy.

6.17. Leukemia (Chronic and Acute)

Leukemia is a type of blood cancer that originates in the bone marrow, leading to the production of abnormal white blood cells. It is broadly classified into **acute** and **chronic** forms, with subtypes based on the affected white blood cells (myeloid or lymphoid).

The two main categories are **acute myeloid leukemia (AML)** and **acute lymphoblastic leukemia (ALL)** for acute leukemias, and **chronic myeloid leukemia (CML)** and **chronic lymphocytic leukemia (CLL)** for chronic leukemias.

6.17.1. Screening for Leukemia

Routine **screening** for leukemia is not recommended in the general population, as there are no established screening protocols, and most leukemias present with clinical symptoms rather than being detected during screening. **NCCN guidelines** do not recommend population-wide screening; however, individuals with certain risk factors or genetic predispositions may require closer monitoring.

High-Risk Populations

Although population-based screening is not feasible, individuals at higher risk due to environmental exposures, genetic predisposition, or prior therapies may benefit from regular health checks and blood work.

- **Genetic Syndromes**: Patients with **Down syndrome, Fanconi anemia, Li-Fraumeni syndrome**, or **Bloom syndrome** are at increased risk of developing leukemia, particularly **AML** and **ALL**. These patients require close surveillance for signs of hematologic abnormalities.
- **Previous Chemotherapy or Radiation**: Individuals who have undergone **chemotherapy** or **radiation therapy** for other cancers are at a higher risk of developing **secondary leukemia**. Regular blood tests (e.g., **complete blood count, CBC**) and monitoring may be advisable.
- **Environmental Exposures**: People with exposure to **benzene, radiation**, or other toxic chemicals may also benefit from more frequent monitoring.

Laboratory Testing

Although routine screening is not performed, certain laboratory tests may raise suspicion of leukemia in at-risk populations or symptomatic patients:

- **Complete Blood Count (CBC)**: A **CBC** with differential can help identify abnormal white blood cell counts, anemia, or thrombocytopenia, which are common in leukemia.
- **Peripheral Blood Smear**: Abnormalities in the size, shape, or number of white blood cells may raise suspicion of leukemia and prompt further testing.
- **Bone Marrow Biopsy**: If leukemia is suspected based on blood tests, a **bone marrow biopsy** is the definitive test for diagnosis, allowing for cytogenetic and molecular analysis of leukemia cells.

6.17.2. Risk Factors for Leukemia

Several factors increase the risk of developing both **acute** and **chronic leukemia**. These risk factors can be genetic, environmental, or related to previous therapies.

Genetic Predisposition

- **Inherited Syndromes**: Certain genetic syndromes, such as **Down syndrome**, significantly increase the risk of developing leukemia, particularly **AML** and **ALL**. Studies show that children with Down syndrome have a **10-20 fold increased risk** of developing leukemia compared to the general population.
- **Family History**: While most leukemia cases are sporadic, a family history of leukemia may increase the risk, particularly for **chronic lymphocytic leukemia (CLL)**. A study by **Goldin et al. (2012)** found that individuals with a first-degree relative with CLL had a **2-4 fold higher risk** of developing the disease.

Environmental Exposures

- **Radiation**: Exposure to high levels of **radiation**, either through environmental exposure (e.g., nuclear disasters) or medical treatment (e.g., radiotherapy), significantly increases the risk of developing leukemia, particularly **acute leukemia**.
- **Chemical Exposure**: Prolonged exposure to **benzene**, a chemical found in industrial settings and some household products, is strongly associated with an increased risk of **AML**.
- **Chemotherapy**: Patients who have undergone **chemotherapy** with alkylating agents or **topoisomerase II inhibitors** for other cancers are at higher risk of developing **secondary leukemia**, particularly AML. This is commonly seen 5-10 years after treatment.

Age and Gender

- **Age**: The risk of leukemia varies with age. **ALL** is most common in children, while **AML** occurs most frequently in older adults. **CML** and **CLL** primarily affect adults, with CLL being the most common leukemia in the elderly.
- **Gender**: Males have a slightly higher risk of developing leukemia than females, with certain subtypes, such as **CLL**, being more prevalent in men.

6.17.3. Treatment of Leukemia: NCCN Guidelines

Treatment for leukemia depends on the subtype (acute vs. chronic), age of the patient, molecular characteristics, and the stage of the disease. The **NCCN guidelines** offer detailed recommendations for the management of each leukemia subtype, incorporating chemotherapy, targeted therapies, immunotherapy, and stem cell transplantation.

Acute Myeloid Leukemia (AML)

AML is an aggressive form of leukemia that requires prompt treatment. The treatment strategy involves **induction chemotherapy** followed by **consolidation therapy**.

- **Induction Chemotherapy**: The goal of induction therapy is to achieve **complete remission** (CR) by reducing the leukemia burden in the bone marrow. The standard induction regimen is **"7+3"** (cytarabine for 7 days and an anthracycline, usually

daunorubicin or idarubicin, for 3 days). A study by **Döhner et al. (2017)** demonstrated that **7+3** remains a cornerstone of AML therapy.
- **Consolidation Therapy**: After achieving remission, patients undergo consolidation therapy to eliminate any residual disease. For younger patients, this often involves high-dose cytarabine. For high-risk patients, **allogeneic stem cell transplantation** is the preferred option.
- **Targeted Therapies**: In recent years, targeted therapies have been developed for patients with specific mutations:
    - **FLT3 inhibitors** (e.g., midostaurin) are recommended for patients with **FLT3 mutations** based on the results of the **RATIFY trial**, which showed that midostaurin improved overall survival when added to standard induction therapy.
    - **IDH1/IDH2 inhibitors** (e.g., ivosidenib, enasidenib) are used for patients with **IDH1/IDH2 mutations**.

Acute Lymphoblastic Leukemia (ALL)

ALL treatment involves intensive **chemotherapy** regimens aimed at achieving remission and preventing central nervous system (CNS) involvement.

- **Induction Therapy**: The backbone of ALL treatment includes **multi-agent chemotherapy**, typically involving vincristine, prednisone, and an anthracycline. Pediatric regimens are adapted for adults with ALL due to the better outcomes observed with these protocols.
- **CNS Prophylaxis**: Given the risk of CNS involvement in ALL, patients receive **intrathecal chemotherapy** (e.g., methotrexate or cytarabine) as part of their treatment.
- **Philadelphia Chromosome-Positive ALL (Ph+ ALL)**: For patients with **Ph+ ALL**, the addition of **tyrosine kinase inhibitors (TKIs)** such as **imatinib** or **dasatinib** to chemotherapy has become standard of care. The **GRAALL-2005 study** demonstrated improved outcomes when TKIs were combined with chemotherapy.
- **Stem Cell Transplantation**: For patients with high-risk disease or those who relapse, **allogeneic stem cell transplantation** is recommended.

Chronic Myeloid Leukemia (CML)

CML is characterized by the presence of the **Philadelphia chromosome** (BCR-ABL fusion gene) and is primarily treated with **tyrosine kinase inhibitors (TKIs)**.

- **TKIs**: The introduction of TKIs, such as **imatinib**, **dasatinib**, and **nilotinib**, has transformed CML into a manageable chronic disease. The **IRIS trial** demonstrated that **imatinib** led to high rates of **complete cytogenetic response** and **overall survival**. Subsequent TKIs have been developed with improved potency and safety profiles.
- **Monitoring Response**: Treatment is monitored using **molecular response** (BCR-ABL transcript levels). Patients who achieve a **major molecular response (MMR)** have excellent long-term outcomes.

- **Stem Cell Transplantation**: Allogeneic stem cell transplantation is reserved for patients who are resistant to TKIs or progress to **blast crisis**.

Chronic Lymphocytic Leukemia (CLL)

CLL is often indolent and may not require treatment immediately upon diagnosis. The decision to treat is based on the patient's symptoms and disease progression.

- **Watchful Waiting**: For asymptomatic patients with early-stage CLL, **watchful waiting** is often recommended. Treatment is initiated if patients develop symptoms such as lymphadenopathy, cytopenias, or rapid disease progression.
- **First-Line Therapy**: For patients requiring treatment, **BTK inhibitors** such as **ibrutinib** or **acalabrutinib** are commonly used, particularly in patients with **unfavorable genetic markers** (e.g., **del(17p)** or **TP53 mutation**). The **RESONATE trial** demonstrated that ibrutinib significantly improved **progression-free survival** compared to ofatumumab in relapsed CLL.
- **Venetoclax and Rituximab**: The combination of **venetoclax** (a BCL-2 inhibitor) and **rituximab** is also approved for patients with relapsed/refractory CLL. The **MURANO trial** showed that venetoclax plus rituximab improved **overall survival** in relapsed CLL.
- **Chimeric Antigen Receptor (CAR) T-Cell Therapy**: For patients with relapsed/refractory CLL who fail multiple lines of therapy, **CAR-T cell therapy** is being explored, although it is more commonly used in aggressive lymphomas.

6.17.4. Latest Advances in Leukemia Treatment

Significant advances in **targeted therapy**, **immunotherapy**, and **genomic profiling** have improved outcomes for patients with both acute and chronic leukemias.

CAR-T Cell Therapy

CAR-T cell therapy has shown promising results in **relapsed/refractory ALL** and **CLL**. **Tisagenlecleucel**, a CAR-T therapy, was approved for pediatric and young adult patients with **relapsed/refractory ALL**, achieving high response rates in clinical trials. **CAR-T therapies** are also being explored in CLL with ongoing studies showing encouraging results.

Venetoclax in AML

Venetoclax, a BCL-2 inhibitor, in combination with **azacitidine** or **decitabine**, has emerged as an effective treatment for **elderly patients with AML** who are ineligible for intensive chemotherapy. The **VIALE-A trial** demonstrated that venetoclax plus azacitidine improved **overall survival** compared to azacitidine alone in this patient population.

Minimal Residual Disease (MRD) Testing

The use of **minimal residual disease (MRD)** testing is becoming increasingly important in both **ALL** and **AML** to guide treatment decisions and assess prognosis. MRD negativity is associated with better outcomes and may influence decisions regarding the need for further therapy or stem cell transplantation.

6.18. Multiple Myeloma

Multiple myeloma (MM) is a hematologic malignancy characterized by the clonal proliferation of plasma cells, which produce monoclonal immunoglobulins (M-protein) leading to bone marrow infiltration, bone destruction, and organ damage.

It is the second most common hematologic cancer after non-Hodgkin lymphoma. With recent advances in **targeted therapies** and **immunotherapy**, survival rates for multiple myeloma have significantly improved.

6.18.1. Screening for Multiple Myeloma

There are currently no routine **screening programs** for multiple myeloma in asymptomatic individuals, as the disease is relatively rare, and no specific screening tests are available for the general population. However, for individuals at high risk or with early signs of the disease, certain tests may aid in early detection.

Screening in High-Risk Populations

While screening is not recommended for the general population, individuals with precursor conditions such as **monoclonal gammopathy of undetermined significance (MGUS)** or **smoldering myeloma** require closer monitoring, as these conditions can progress to symptomatic multiple myeloma.

- **MGUS**: A premalignant plasma cell disorder, MGUS is characterized by the presence of monoclonal protein in the blood without the clinical features of multiple myeloma. Approximately **1% of patients** with MGUS progress to multiple myeloma annually. The **NCCN guidelines** recommend that patients with MGUS undergo annual monitoring with **serum protein electrophoresis (SPEP), immunofixation,** and **free light chain assays**.
- **Smoldering Multiple Myeloma**: This is an intermediate stage between MGUS and symptomatic myeloma. Patients with smoldering myeloma are at a higher risk of progression and should be monitored every 3-6 months with **imaging** and **laboratory tests** to detect signs of progression to symptomatic disease.

Early Detection Through Biomarkers

While routine screening is not recommended, early signs of multiple myeloma, such as **anemia, hypercalcemia, elevated serum creatinine,** or **bone lesions**, often prompt further diagnostic workup. **SPEP, urine protein electrophoresis (UPEP),** and **serum free light chain assay** are used to detect monoclonal proteins associated with myeloma.

- **Imaging**: Low-dose whole-body CT scans, PET-CT, and MRI can identify **bone lesions** or other structural changes associated with multiple myeloma

6.18.2. Risk Factors for Multiple Myeloma

Several risk factors contribute to the development of multiple myeloma, including genetic predisposition, environmental exposures, and certain pre-existing conditions.

Genetic and Familial Factors

- **Family History**: Having a first-degree relative with multiple myeloma increases the risk of developing the disease. **Goldin et al. (2014)** showed that individuals with a family history of hematologic malignancies have a **2-3 fold increased risk** of developing multiple myeloma.
- **Race**: African Americans have nearly **twice the risk** of developing multiple myeloma compared to Caucasians, suggesting that genetic factors play a significant role in disease susceptibility.

Environmental and Occupational Exposures

- **Radiation Exposure**: Exposure to high doses of radiation, as seen in survivors of nuclear disasters, increases the risk of multiple myeloma.
- **Chemical Exposure**: Prolonged exposure to certain chemicals, such as **benzene** and **pesticides**, has been linked to an increased risk of multiple myeloma.

Monoclonal Gammopathy of Undetermined Significance (MGUS)

MGUS is a significant risk factor for developing multiple myeloma. **Approximately 1% of individuals with MGUS** progress to multiple myeloma annually, and the risk of progression depends on factors such as the level of **monoclonal protein**, the **IgM subtype**, and the **serum free light chain ratio**.

Age and Gender

Multiple myeloma is primarily a disease of older adults, with a median age of diagnosis around **69 years**. It is more common in **men** than in women.

6.18.3. Treatment of Multiple Myeloma: NCCN Guidelines

The treatment of multiple myeloma is tailored to the stage of the disease, the patient's performance status, and the presence of high-risk features, such as specific genetic mutations (e.g., **del(17p)**). The **NCCN guidelines** outline a comprehensive approach that incorporates **chemotherapy, immunotherapy, targeted therapies, stem cell transplantation**, and **supportive care**.

Induction Therapy for Transplant-Eligible Patients

For younger, fit patients who are eligible for **autologous stem cell transplantation (ASCT)**, treatment typically begins with **induction therapy** aimed at reducing tumor burden before transplant.

- **Triplet Regimens**: The most commonly used induction regimens include **bortezomib (a proteasome inhibitor), lenalidomide (an immunomodulatory drug, IMiD), and dexamethasone** (VRd regimen). The **IFM 2009 study** showed that using VRd as induction therapy significantly improved **progression-free survival (PFS)** and **overall survival (OS)** in transplant-eligible patients.
- **ASCT**: After induction therapy, patients undergo **high-dose chemotherapy** with melphalan followed by **ASCT**, which remains the standard of care for eligible patients. Studies like **Attal et al. (2015)** have demonstrated the benefits of ASCT in prolonging **remission**.

Induction Therapy for Transplant-Ineligible Patients

For older or frail patients who are not candidates for stem cell transplantation, similar **triplet regimens** are used, though the doses are adjusted to reduce toxicity.

- **VRd-Lite**: A modified, lower-dose version of the VRd regimen is often used in transplant-ineligible patients. In the **SWOG S0777 trial**, patients receiving VRd demonstrated improved **PFS** and **OS** compared to lenalidomide and dexamethasone alone.

Maintenance Therapy

Maintenance therapy with **lenalidomide** or **bortezomib** after induction therapy and ASCT has been shown to prolong **PFS** and **OS**. The **CALGB 100104 trial** demonstrated that lenalidomide maintenance significantly extended **overall survival** compared to observation alone.

Relapsed/Refractory Disease

For patients with **relapsed or refractory multiple myeloma**, a range of therapies are available depending on previous treatments and genetic features.

- **Daratumumab**: A **monoclonal antibody** targeting **CD38**, daratumumab has shown significant efficacy in relapsed myeloma. The **CASTOR trial** demonstrated that combining daratumumab with bortezomib and dexamethasone improved **PFS** in patients with relapsed disease.
- **Carfilzomib**: A next-generation proteasome inhibitor, **carfilzomib** is effective in patients who relapse after treatment with bortezomib. The **ENDEAVOR trial** showed that carfilzomib improved PFS compared to bortezomib in patients with relapsed myeloma.
- **Venetoclax**: For patients with **t(11;14) translocations**, the BCL-2 inhibitor **venetoclax** has demonstrated efficacy in combination with dexamethasone or other agents.

6.18.4. Latest Advances in Multiple Myeloma Treatment

Significant advances in **immunotherapy**, **targeted therapies**, and **CAR-T cell therapies** have transformed the treatment landscape for multiple myeloma.

CAR-T Cell Therapy

Chimeric Antigen Receptor (CAR) T-cell therapy has revolutionized the treatment of relapsed/refractory multiple myeloma. **Idecabtagene vicleucel (ide-cel)**, which targets **BCMA (B-cell maturation antigen)** on myeloma cells, was approved by the FDA for patients with heavily pretreated disease.

- The **KarMMa trial** showed that ide-cel achieved high response rates in patients with relapsed or refractory myeloma, with many patients achieving durable remissions.

Bispecific Antibodies

Bispecific antibodies are designed to engage both **T-cells** and **myeloma cells**, facilitating an immune attack against the cancer. **Teclistamab**, a bispecific antibody targeting **BCMA**, has shown promising results in early trials, with high response rates in relapsed myeloma patients.

Selinexor

Selinexor, a selective inhibitor of nuclear export, is a novel oral agent approved for relapsed/refractory multiple myeloma. In the **STORM trial**, selinexor combined with dexamethasone achieved responses in patients who had exhausted standard treatment options.

Venetoclax for t(11;14)

For patients with **t(11;14) translocations**, the BCL-2 inhibitor **venetoclax** has shown significant activity. In combination with bortezomib, venetoclax improves PFS in patients with this specific genetic mutation.

6.19. Endometrial Cancer

Endometrial cancer, the most common gynecologic malignancy in developed countries, arises from the lining of the uterus (endometrium). The majority of cases are diagnosed at an early stage due to the common presentation of postmenopausal bleeding, which allows for favorable outcomes.

6.19.1. Screening for Endometrial Cancer

There are currently no routine screening programs for endometrial cancer in the general population. Most cases are diagnosed following the onset of symptoms, such as **abnormal uterine bleeding**, especially in postmenopausal women. However, for high-risk populations, such as women with **hereditary cancer syndromes**, screening and preventive measures are essential.

High-Risk Populations

While routine population-wide screening is not recommended, women with certain risk factors, particularly those with **Lynch syndrome** (hereditary non-polyposis colorectal cancer, HNPCC), should undergo regular monitoring for endometrial cancer.

- **Lynch Syndrome**: Women with **Lynch syndrome** have a significantly increased lifetime risk (up to **40-60%**) of developing endometrial cancer. The **NCCN guidelines** recommend **annual endometrial biopsy** starting at age 30-35 for women with Lynch syndrome. **Hysterectomy** may also be considered as a preventive measure after childbearing is complete.
- **Tamoxifen Use**: Women taking **tamoxifen** for breast cancer prevention or treatment are at increased risk for endometrial cancer due to its estrogen agonist effects on the uterus. These women should be monitored closely for symptoms of abnormal bleeding.

Diagnostic Tests for Symptomatic Women

In symptomatic women, especially those presenting with **postmenopausal bleeding**, several diagnostic tools are used to detect or confirm endometrial cancer:

- **Transvaginal Ultrasound (TVUS)**: TVUS is commonly used to measure **endometrial thickness**. An endometrial thickness of less than **4 mm** in postmenopausal women with bleeding is generally considered reassuring, while a thicker endometrium may warrant further investigation.
- **Endometrial Biopsy**: Endometrial biopsy is the gold standard for diagnosing endometrial cancer in women with abnormal uterine bleeding. It is a simple and minimally invasive procedure with high diagnostic accuracy.
- **Hysteroscopy**: If endometrial biopsy is inconclusive or if abnormal findings are noted, **hysteroscopy** with directed biopsy can be performed for further evaluation.

6.19.2. Risk Factors for Endometrial Cancer

Several **risk factors** have been identified for the development of endometrial cancer. The most significant are related to **hormonal imbalances**, particularly unopposed estrogen exposure, and genetic predispositions.

Hormonal Factors

- **Unopposed Estrogen**: **Excess estrogen exposure** without opposition from progesterone is the most significant risk factor for endometrial cancer. Conditions such as **obesity, polycystic ovary syndrome (PCOS), estrogen-only hormone replacement therapy**, and **late menopause** all increase the risk by prolonging or increasing estrogen exposure.

- **Obesity**: Obesity is a major risk factor for endometrial cancer, as adipose tissue converts androgens into estrogen, leading to higher circulating estrogen levels. Studies show that obese women have a **2-4 fold increased risk** of endometrial cancer compared to women with normal weight.
- **Tamoxifen**: While **tamoxifen** is used as a treatment and preventive agent for breast cancer, it acts as an estrogen agonist in the uterus, increasing the risk of endometrial cancer, particularly with prolonged use.

Genetic Factors

- **Lynch Syndrome**: As mentioned earlier, women with **Lynch syndrome** are at a significantly increased risk of developing endometrial cancer. Genetic mutations in **MLH1, MSH2, MSH6**, or **PMS2** drive the development of this syndrome.

Age and Reproductive Factors

- **Age**: Endometrial cancer is primarily a disease of **postmenopausal women**, with the majority of cases diagnosed after the age of 50.
- **Nulliparity**: Women who have never given birth have a higher risk of endometrial cancer, possibly due to longer periods of unopposed estrogen exposure.
- **Early Menarche and Late Menopause**: Women who experience **early menarche** or **late menopause** are at increased risk due to a longer lifetime exposure to estrogen.

Diabetes and Hypertension

Women with **diabetes** and **hypertension** are at increased risk of developing endometrial cancer, likely due to overlapping risk factors with obesity and metabolic syndrome.

6.19.3. Treatment of Endometrial Cancer: NCCN Guidelines

The treatment of endometrial cancer depends on the stage at diagnosis, the patient's performance status, and the histological subtype of the tumor. The **NCCN guidelines** provide clear recommendations for the management of early, advanced, and recurrent endometrial cancer.

Surgery

Surgery is the mainstay of treatment for endometrial cancer and is generally curative for early-stage disease. The standard surgical procedure is a **total hysterectomy** with bilateral salpingo-oophorectomy (BSO).

- **Sentinel Lymph Node Biopsy**: In patients with early-stage disease, **sentinel lymph node biopsy** has been shown to reduce morbidity compared to full lymphadenectomy while maintaining accurate staging. Studies like **SENTI-ENDO** demonstrated that sentinel node mapping is safe and effective for staging.

- **Lymph Node Dissection**: Lymph node dissection is performed selectively in patients with **high-risk features** (e.g., higher-grade tumors or deep myometrial invasion) to assess for metastasis.

Adjuvant Therapy

Adjuvant therapy, including **radiation** and **chemotherapy**, is recommended based on the stage and risk factors for recurrence.

- **Radiation Therapy**: For **intermediate- and high-risk patients**, radiation therapy is recommended postoperatively. The **PORTEC-2 trial** showed that **vaginal brachytherapy** is effective in reducing local recurrence with fewer side effects compared to external beam radiation therapy (EBRT) in patients with early-stage, high-risk disease.
- **Chemotherapy**: For patients with advanced-stage or high-risk disease (e.g., serous carcinoma or clear cell carcinoma), **systemic chemotherapy** is often recommended. Common regimens include **carboplatin** and **paclitaxel**. The **GOG-209 trial** found that the combination of carboplatin and paclitaxel was as effective as other chemotherapy regimens and better tolerated.

Hormonal Therapy

For patients with **low-grade, hormone receptor-positive tumors**, hormonal therapy can be an effective treatment option, especially in those who are not surgical candidates or who wish to preserve fertility.

- **Progestins**: Progestin therapy (e.g., **medroxyprogesterone acetate** or **megestrol acetate**) is commonly used for **early-stage**, low-risk patients who wish to preserve fertility. Hormonal therapy is also used in advanced or recurrent disease that expresses hormone receptors.

Treatment of Advanced and Recurrent Disease

For advanced or recurrent endometrial cancer, multimodal treatment approaches are often necessary:

- **Chemotherapy and Radiation**: In advanced cases, **chemotherapy** with **carboplatin and paclitaxel**, sometimes combined with **radiation therapy**, is the standard of care.
- **Immunotherapy**: Immunotherapy has emerged as a promising treatment option for patients with **advanced endometrial cancer**, particularly those with **microsatellite instability-high (MSI-H)** or **mismatch repair-deficient (dMMR)** tumors. **Pembrolizumab**, an anti-PD-1 monoclonal antibody, has been FDA-approved for **MSI-H** endometrial cancer based on results from the **KEYNOTE-158 trial**, which demonstrated durable responses in heavily pretreated patients.

6.19.4. Latest Advances in Endometrial Cancer Treatment

Recent advances in the treatment of endometrial cancer have focused on **targeted therapies** and **immunotherapy**. These therapies are offering new hope, particularly for patients with advanced or recurrent disease.

Targeted Therapies

Targeted therapies are becoming increasingly important in the management of high-risk or advanced endometrial cancer:

- **Pembrolizumab and Lenvatinib**: The combination of **pembrolizumab** (a PD-1 inhibitor) and **lenvatinib** (a tyrosine kinase inhibitor) has shown promising results in patients with **advanced, microsatellite-stable (MSS) endometrial cancer** who have progressed after prior therapies. The **KEYNOTE-775 trial** demonstrated that this combination significantly improved **progression-free survival (PFS)** and **overall survival (OS)** compared to chemotherapy.

PARP Inhibitors

PARP inhibitors, such as **olaparib** and **niraparib**, are being investigated for use in endometrial cancer, particularly in patients with DNA repair deficiencies, such as those with **BRCA mutations** or **homologous recombination deficiency (HRD)**.

Hormonal Therapy in Combination with Targeted Therapies

New trials are investigating combinations of **hormonal therapy** with targeted agents like **CDK4/6 inhibitors** (e.g., palbociclib) to improve outcomes in patients with hormone receptor-positive endometrial cancer.

6.20. Head and Neck Cancers

Head and neck cancer (HNC) encompasses a diverse group of malignancies that arise from the mucosal surfaces of the oral cavity, pharynx, larynx, nasal cavity, paranasal sinuses, and salivary glands. The majority of these cancers are **squamous cell carcinomas (HNSCC)**, which are linked to **tobacco use, alcohol consumption**, and **human papillomavirus (HPV)** infection.

Due to its aggressive nature and the complexity of the anatomic regions involved, treatment of head and neck cancer requires a multidisciplinary approach. Advances in **immunotherapy** and **targeted therapies** have transformed the management of advanced disease.

6.20.1. Screening for Head and Neck Cancer

There are no established routine screening programs for head and neck cancer in the general population. However, screening efforts are more targeted toward **high-risk individuals**, such as those with a history of **tobacco** and **alcohol** use or **HPV** infection.

Screening for High-Risk Populations

High-risk individuals, particularly long-term smokers, heavy drinkers, or those with a history of **HPV-associated oral infections**, may benefit from close monitoring for early signs of head and neck cancer.

- **Oral Screening Exams**: Routine **oral exams** performed by primary care physicians or dentists can help detect early signs of cancer in high-risk individuals. Visual inspection and palpation of the oral cavity, including the tongue, gums, and throat, can identify early lesions or changes in mucosal tissue.
- **HPV Screening**: Screening for **HPV** is not routinely recommended for the general population. However, individuals with HPV-related risk factors may benefit from testing. Studies have shown that **HPV-positive oropharyngeal cancer** has distinct clinical features and better prognosis compared to HPV-negative cancers.

Diagnostic Testing for Symptomatic Patients

For patients presenting with symptoms such as **persistent hoarseness, sore throat, difficulty swallowing, lumps in the neck**, or **unexplained weight loss**, diagnostic workup is essential.

- **Endoscopy**: Direct **laryngoscopy** or **nasopharyngoscopy** can visualize tumors in the upper aerodigestive tract. It is an essential tool in the initial evaluation of head and neck cancer.
- **Imaging**: Imaging studies, including **CT**, **MRI**, and **PET scans**, are critical in staging the disease and determining the extent of local and distant involvement. **PET-CT** is particularly useful in detecting distant metastases and assessing treatment response.
- **Biopsy**: A tissue biopsy of any suspicious lesion is required for a definitive diagnosis. Biopsy methods can include **fine-needle aspiration (FNA)** for neck masses or **direct biopsy** of visible lesions during endoscopy.

6.20.2. Risk Factors for Head and Neck Cancer

Several well-established risk factors contribute to the development of head and neck cancer. The most common are **tobacco use, alcohol consumption**, and **HPV infection**.

Tobacco and Alcohol Use

- **Tobacco Use**: **Tobacco smoking** remains the most significant risk factor for head and neck cancer. Smokers are estimated to have a **10-20 times higher risk** of developing head and neck cancer compared to non-smokers. The synergistic effect of **tobacco and alcohol** use further increases this risk. Even **second-hand smoke** exposure has been linked to an increased risk of developing HNC.

- **Alcohol Use**: **Heavy alcohol consumption** is another major risk factor. Alcohol acts synergistically with tobacco to increase the risk of **oral**, **oropharyngeal**, and **laryngeal** cancers. Alcohol alone can damage the mucosa, making it more susceptible to carcinogens in tobacco.

Human Papillomavirus (HPV) Infection

- **HPV Infection**: HPV, particularly the **HPV-16** subtype, is strongly associated with **oropharyngeal squamous cell carcinoma** (OPSCC). The incidence of HPV-related oropharyngeal cancers has risen sharply in recent years, particularly in younger, non-smoking individuals. **HPV-positive OPSCC** tends to have a better prognosis than HPV-negative cancers. The **PATRICIA trial** demonstrated that **HPV vaccination** significantly reduces the risk of oral and genital HPV infections.

Other Risk Factors

- **Poor Oral Hygiene**: Poor oral hygiene and chronic irritation from ill-fitting dentures or dental conditions may contribute to an increased risk of oral cancers.
- **Occupational Exposure**: Workers exposed to certain chemicals, including **asbestos**, **wood dust**, and **industrial solvents**, are at increased risk of head and neck cancers, particularly **nasopharyngeal carcinoma**.
- **Epstein-Barr Virus (EBV)**: EBV is associated with **nasopharyngeal carcinoma**. In regions such as Southeast Asia, where nasopharyngeal carcinoma is more common, EBV plays a significant etiologic role.

6.20.3. Treatment of Head and Neck Cancer: NCCN Guidelines

The treatment of head and neck cancer is determined by the **tumor site**, **stage**, **histology**, and the patient's overall health status. The **NCCN guidelines** recommend a **multidisciplinary approach** that combines **surgery**, **radiation therapy**, **chemotherapy**, and, in some cases, **immunotherapy**. The goal of treatment is to achieve local and regional control of the disease while preserving function.

Surgery

Surgery is the cornerstone of treatment for early-stage and resectable tumors. The type of surgery depends on the tumor's location and size.

- **Transoral Robotic Surgery (TORS)**: For selected cases of oropharyngeal cancer, particularly **HPV-positive tumors**, **transoral robotic surgery (TORS)** allows for minimally invasive resection with excellent functional outcomes. Studies such as **Mehanna et al. (2016)** have shown that TORS is effective in treating early-stage oropharyngeal cancers with reduced morbidity.
- **Neck Dissection**: If there is lymph node involvement, **neck dissection** is performed to remove metastatic lymph nodes. Depending on the extent of disease, this may be a **selective**, **modified radical**, or **radical neck dissection**.

Radiation Therapy

Radiation therapy, either alone or combined with surgery or chemotherapy, is a key component of treatment for head and neck cancer. **Intensity-modulated radiation therapy (IMRT)** allows for precise targeting of tumors, minimizing damage to surrounding tissues and reducing side effects.

- **Postoperative Radiation**: For patients with high-risk features after surgery (e.g., positive margins, extracapsular nodal extension), **postoperative radiation therapy (PORT)** is recommended.
- **Definitive Radiation**: For patients with inoperable or unresectable tumors, radiation therapy with or without chemotherapy can be curative. **IMRT** has become the standard radiation technique for these patients due to its ability to spare healthy tissues, particularly in the **oropharynx** and **larynx**.

Chemotherapy

Chemotherapy is used as part of **concurrent chemoradiation** or as **palliative therapy** for advanced or metastatic disease.

- **Platinum-based Chemotherapy**: **Cisplatin** is the most commonly used chemotherapeutic agent, particularly in combination with radiation therapy for **locally advanced disease**. Studies like **Bonner et al. (2006)** demonstrated that adding **cisplatin** to radiation therapy improves **overall survival** in patients with locally advanced HNSCC.

Immunotherapy

Immunotherapy has emerged as a promising treatment for recurrent or metastatic head and neck cancer, particularly for patients whose tumors express **PD-L1**.

- **Checkpoint Inhibitors**: **Pembrolizumab** and **nivolumab**, both **PD-1 inhibitors**, have been approved for patients with recurrent or metastatic HNSCC. The **KEYNOTE-048 trial** demonstrated that **pembrolizumab** significantly improved **overall survival** compared to standard chemotherapy in patients with PD-L1-positive recurrent or metastatic HNSCC.
- **Nivolumab**: The **CheckMate 141 trial** showed that **nivolumab** improved **overall survival** in patients with platinum-refractory recurrent or metastatic head and neck cancer compared to standard therapy.

Targeted Therapy

Cetuximab, a **monoclonal antibody targeting EGFR**, is used in combination with radiation therapy or chemotherapy in patients with advanced HNSCC. The **EXTREME trial** demonstrated that **cetuximab** in combination with platinum-based chemotherapy improved overall survival in patients with recurrent or metastatic HNSCC.

Palliative Care

For patients with advanced, inoperable disease or those who have failed multiple lines of treatment, palliative care focuses on **symptom management** and improving **quality of life**. **Radiation therapy** and **chemotherapy** may be used for **pain relief**, **dysphagia**, and other symptoms of tumor progression.

6.20.4. Latest Advances in Head and Neck Cancer Treatment

The treatment landscape for head and neck cancer has evolved significantly with the introduction of **immunotherapy, targeted therapies**, and **minimally invasive surgical techniques**.

Immunotherapy

The rise of **checkpoint inhibitors** has changed the treatment paradigm for patients with **recurrent or metastatic disease**.

- **KEYNOTE-048 Trial**: This trial demonstrated that **pembrolizumab** improved **overall survival** in patients with PD-L1-positive recurrent or metastatic HNSCC compared to standard chemotherapy. **Pembrolizumab** has become the first-line therapy for this patient population.
- **CheckMate 141 Trial: Nivolumab**, another PD-1 inhibitor, showed improved **overall survival** in patients with **platinum-refractory recurrent or metastatic HNSCC** compared to standard therapy.

Targeted Therapy

Cetuximab, an **EGFR inhibitor**, has been used successfully in combination with radiation and chemotherapy. Ongoing research is exploring **combination therapies** that include both **targeted agents** and **immunotherapies** for advanced head and neck cancers.

De-escalation Strategies for HPV-Positive Cancers

Given the improved prognosis of **HPV-positive oropharyngeal cancer**, researchers are exploring **treatment de-escalation strategies** to reduce long-term side effects without compromising efficacy.

- Trials like **ECOG 3311** are investigating the use of reduced doses of radiation and chemotherapy in patients with HPV-positive cancers following surgery to minimize toxicity while maintaining high cure rates.

6.21. Thyroid Cancer

Thyroid cancer arises from the thyroid gland, and it is the most common endocrine malignancy. It is classified into several subtypes, with **papillary thyroid carcinoma (PTC)**

being the most prevalent, followed by **follicular thyroid carcinoma (FTC)**, **medullary thyroid carcinoma (MTC)**, and **anaplastic thyroid carcinoma (ATC)**.

Most thyroid cancers have an excellent prognosis, especially when diagnosed at an early stage. Advances in molecular testing and targeted therapies have led to significant changes in the management of aggressive and advanced thyroid cancers.

6.21.1. Screening for Thyroid Cancer

Routine **screening** for thyroid cancer is not recommended for the general population because thyroid cancer is relatively rare, and the majority of cases are indolent. Additionally, over-diagnosis of small, subclinical thyroid cancers (detected through imaging studies done for unrelated reasons) has become a concern, as many of these cases do not require aggressive treatment.

Screening in High-Risk Populations

While population-wide screening is not recommended, certain high-risk groups may benefit from **targeted screening**. These groups include:

- **Patients with Family History of Thyroid Cancer**: Individuals with a family history of **medullary thyroid carcinoma (MTC)** or familial syndromes (e.g., **multiple endocrine neoplasia type 2, MEN2**) are at increased risk of thyroid cancer. Genetic testing for **RET mutations** is recommended in individuals with MEN2 or familial MTC.
- **Radiation Exposure**: Individuals who have had **radiation exposure** to the head and neck, especially during childhood, are at increased risk of thyroid cancer. Long-term survivors of **childhood cancers** treated with radiation are at higher risk and may require regular monitoring with **neck ultrasound** and **thyroid function tests**.

Diagnostic Workup for Suspected Thyroid Cancer

When thyroid nodules are detected, the workup usually includes the following steps:

- **Thyroid Ultrasound**: **Neck ultrasound** is the primary imaging modality used to evaluate thyroid nodules. Features such as **hypoechogenicity**, **irregular margins**, **microcalcifications**, and **taller-than-wide shape** raise the suspicion of malignancy.
- **Fine Needle Aspiration (FNA) Biopsy**: FNA biopsy is used to evaluate thyroid nodules that are suspicious on ultrasound or larger than **1 cm**. The **Bethesda System for Reporting Thyroid Cytopathology** is used to classify FNA findings into six categories, ranging from benign to malignant.
- **Molecular Testing**: Molecular markers such as **BRAF, RAS, RET/PTC rearrangements**, and **Tert promoter mutations** are increasingly used to assess the risk of malignancy in indeterminate thyroid nodules.

6.21.2. Risk Factors for Thyroid Cancer

Several risk factors contribute to the development of thyroid cancer, including genetic factors, environmental exposures, and certain medical conditions.

Radiation Exposure

- **Radiation** is the most well-established risk factor for thyroid cancer, particularly **papillary thyroid carcinoma (PTC)**. Individuals who were exposed to **ionizing radiation** during childhood, either from medical treatments (e.g., radiation therapy for other cancers) or environmental exposure (e.g., nuclear accidents), have a significantly increased risk of developing thyroid cancer later in life.
- A study by **Ron et al. (1995)** demonstrated that **children exposed to radiation** have a **2-3 fold increased risk** of developing thyroid cancer compared to non-exposed individuals.

Genetic Factors

- **Familial Syndromes**: Thyroid cancer can occur as part of familial cancer syndromes, such as **multiple endocrine neoplasia type 2 (MEN2)**, which is associated with **medullary thyroid carcinoma (MTC)**. Genetic mutations in the **RET proto-oncogene** are common in these patients. Familial **adenomatous polyposis (FAP)** and **Cowden syndrome** are associated with an increased risk of **papillary thyroid carcinoma**.
- **Genetic Mutations**: Somatic mutations in genes such as BRAF (particularly **BRAF V600E**), **RAS**, and **RET/PTC rearrangements** are frequently found in thyroid cancers and are associated with more aggressive disease in certain subtypes.

Gender and Age

- **Gender**: Thyroid cancer is more common in **women**, with a female-to-male ratio of approximately **3:1**. Hormonal factors may play a role in this discrepancy, although the exact mechanism remains unclear.
- **Age**: The incidence of thyroid cancer peaks in individuals aged **30-50 years. Younger age** at diagnosis is generally associated with a better prognosis, except in cases of **anaplastic thyroid carcinoma**.

Iodine Deficiency and Excess

- **Iodine Deficiency**: In regions with **iodine deficiency**, there is an increased incidence of **follicular thyroid carcinoma**. Conversely, **excess iodine intake** can also predispose to thyroid dysfunction and possibly cancer in susceptible individuals.

6.21.3. Treatment of Thyroid Cancer: NCCN Guidelines

The treatment of thyroid cancer is largely determined by the **histological subtype, tumor stage**, and **risk factors**. The **NCCN guidelines** provide detailed recommendations for the management of the most common thyroid cancers, including **papillary, follicular, medullary,** and **anaplastic thyroid carcinoma**.

Surgery

Surgery is the primary treatment for most cases of thyroid cancer, especially for **differentiated thyroid cancers** (i.e., papillary and follicular thyroid carcinoma).

- **Thyroid Lobectomy vs. Total Thyroidectomy**: The extent of surgery depends on the tumor size, location, and presence of metastasis. For tumors smaller than **1 cm** (microcarcinomas), **lobectomy** may be sufficient. However, for larger tumors or those with aggressive features, **total thyroidectomy** is recommended. Studies like **Bilimoria et al. (2007)** showed that **total thyroidectomy** is associated with better outcomes for tumors larger than 1 cm.
- **Lymph Node Dissection**: In cases of **lymph node involvement, central compartment lymph node dissection** is performed. **Prophylactic dissection** is often considered for **high-risk** patients, but it is not routinely recommended for low-risk individuals.

Radioactive Iodine (RAI) Therapy

For **differentiated thyroid cancers** (papillary and follicular), **radioactive iodine (RAI)** therapy is used to ablate residual thyroid tissue or treat metastases after surgery.

- **RAI Ablation**: Postoperative **RAI ablation** is recommended for patients with **high-risk features**, including **large tumors, lymph node metastasis**, or **distant metastasis**. Studies such as **Mazzaferri and Jhiang (1994)** showed that RAI improves outcomes in high-risk patients but is not necessary for low-risk, small tumors.
- **RAI-Refractory Disease**: In patients with **RAI-refractory disease**, who do not respond to RAI therapy, **systemic therapies** such as **targeted kinase inhibitors** may be considered (see below).

Thyroid Hormone Suppression Therapy

After surgery, patients are typically treated with **thyroid hormone suppression therapy** to suppress **thyroid-stimulating hormone (TSH)**, which can stimulate cancer cell growth.

- **Levothyroxine** is used to maintain **low TSH levels** in patients at high risk of recurrence. The **NCCN guidelines** recommend maintaining **TSH suppression** for several years in patients with high-risk features.

Systemic Therapy for Advanced and Refractory Disease

For patients with **metastatic** or **RAI-refractory differentiated thyroid cancer**, systemic therapy is often required.

- **Tyrosine Kinase Inhibitors (TKIs)**: Targeted therapies such as **lenvatinib** and **sorafenib** are used for patients with advanced thyroid cancer. The **SELECT trial** demonstrated that **lenvatinib** significantly improved **progression-free survival (PFS)** in patients with RAI-refractory thyroid cancer compared to placebo.

- **Medullary Thyroid Carcinoma (MTC)**: For patients with advanced or metastatic **medullary thyroid carcinoma**, targeted therapies such as **vandetanib** and **cabozantinib** are FDA-approved. Both agents target the **RET mutation**, commonly found in MTC. The **EXAM trial** showed that **cabozantinib** improved PFS in patients with advanced MTC.
- **Anaplastic Thyroid Carcinoma (ATC)**: ATC is an aggressive subtype with poor prognosis. Treatment is often palliative and includes **surgery**, **chemotherapy**, and **radiation**. For patients with **BRAF V600E mutations**, **dabrafenib** and **trametinib** have been shown to improve outcomes. The **BREAKFAST trial** demonstrated the efficacy of this combination in patients with BRAF-mutated ATC.

6.21.4. Latest Advances in Thyroid Cancer Treatment

Recent advances in **targeted therapy**, **immunotherapy**, and **genetic testing** have transformed the treatment of advanced thyroid cancers, particularly those resistant to conventional therapies.

Targeted Therapy

- **Lenvatinib and Sorafenib**: These **multi-kinase inhibitors** target VEGF, FGFR, and RET pathways and are approved for use in **RAI-refractory differentiated thyroid cancers**. The **SELECT trial** demonstrated that lenvatinib improved **progression-free survival** by nearly 18 months compared to placebo.
- **Vandetanib and Cabozantinib for MTC**: For patients with advanced **medullary thyroid carcinoma**, both **vandetanib** and **cabozantinib** target **RET mutations**. Studies like the **ZETA trial** (vandetanib) and **EXAM trial** (cabozantinib) showed significant improvements in PFS in patients with advanced MTC

Immunotherapy

Immunotherapy is an emerging treatment for **anaplastic thyroid carcinoma (ATC)** and other aggressive thyroid cancers. While not yet standard, immune checkpoint inhibitors such as **pembrolizumab** (anti-PD-1) are being investigated in clinical trials for advanced thyroid cancers.

- Studies like **KEYNOTE-028** demonstrated that **pembrolizumab** shows promise in treating **PD-L1-positive advanced thyroid cancers**, although further trials are needed to confirm its efficacy.

Genetic Testing and Precision Medicine

The use of **molecular testing** to identify mutations such as **BRAF V600E**, **RET/PTC**, and **Tert promoter mutations** allows for **precision medicine** approaches in thyroid cancer treatment.

- The discovery of **BRAF mutations** has revolutionized treatment for **anaplastic thyroid carcinoma** and aggressive **papillary thyroid carcinoma**, as **BRAF inhibitors** like **dabrafenib** and **trametinib** show efficacy in these patients.

References

- Sparano JA, Gray RJ, Makower DF, et al. Adjuvant chemotherapy guided by a 21-gene expression assay in breast cancer. *N Engl J Med*. 2018;379(2):111-121.
- Reck M, Rodríguez-Abreu D, Robinson AG, et al. Pembrolizumab versus chemotherapy for PD-L1–positive non–small-cell lung cancer. *N Engl J Med*. 2016;375(19):1823-1833.
- Le DT, Durham JN, Smith KN, et al. Mismatch repair deficiency predicts response of solid tumors to PD-1 blockade. *Science*. 2017;357(6349):409-413.
- Robson M, Im SA, Senkus E, et al. Olaparib for metastatic breast cancer in patients with a germline BRCA mutation. *N Engl J Med*. 2017;377(6):523-533.
- Younes A, Connors JM, Park SI, et al. Brentuximab vedotin combined with chemotherapy for stage III or IV Hodgkin's lymphoma. *N Engl J Med*. 2013;368(8):679-688.
- Maude SL, Laetsch TW, Buechner J, et al. Tisagenlecleucel in children and young adults with B-cell lymphoblastic leukemia. *N Engl J Med*. 2018;378(5):439-448.
- NCCN Guidelines: National Comprehensive Cancer Network. Breast Cancer (Version 4.2023).
- Oncotype DX Study: Sparano JA, et al. TAILORx trial. "Adjuvant Chemotherapy Guided by a 21-Gene Expression Assay in Breast Cancer." *New England Journal of Medicine*, 2018.
- PARP Inhibitors Study: Robson M, et al. OlympiAD trial. "Olaparib for Metastatic Breast Cancer in Patients with a Germline BRCA Mutation." *New England Journal of Medicine*, 2017.
- NCCN Guidelines: National Comprehensive Cancer Network. Non-Small Cell Lung Cancer (NSCLC) (Version 4.2023); Small Cell Lung Cancer (SCLC) (Version 2.2023).
- Immunotherapy Study: Reck M, et al. KEYNOTE-024 trial. "Pembrolizumab versus Chemotherapy for PD-L1–Positive NSCLC." *New England Journal of Medicine*, 2016.
- NCCN Guidelines: National Comprehensive Cancer Network. Colon Cancer (Version 4.2023); Rectal Cancer (Version 2.2023).
- FOLFOX Chemotherapy Study: André T, et al. "Oxaliplatin, Fluorouracil, and Leucovorin as Adjuvant Treatment for Colon Cancer." *New England Journal of Medicine*, 2004.
- Immunotherapy for MSI-H Tumors: Le DT, et al. KEYNOTE-177 trial. "Pembrolizumab versus Chemotherapy for MSI-H Colorectal Cancer." *New England Journal of Medicine*, 2020.
- NCCN Guidelines: National Comprehensive Cancer Network. Prostate Cancer (Version 2.2024).
- Castration-Resistant Study: Smith MR, et al. SPARTAN trial. "Apalutamide Treatment and Metastasis-Free Survival in Prostate Cancer." *New England Journal of Medicine*, 2018.

- NCCN Guidelines: National Comprehensive Cancer Network. Cervical Cancer (Version 1.2024).
- Immunotherapy Study: Tewari KS, et al. KEYNOTE-826 trial. "Pembrolizumab in Cervical Cancer." *New England Journal of Medicine*, 2021.
- NCCN Guidelines: National Comprehensive Cancer Network. Ovarian Cancer (Version 3.2024).
- PARP Inhibitors Study: Moore K, et al. SOLO-1 trial. "Olaparib for Newly Diagnosed Advanced Ovarian Cancer." *New England Journal of Medicine*, 2018.
- NCCN Guidelines: National Comprehensive Cancer Network. Pancreatic Adenocarcinoma (Version 2.2024).
- FOLFIRINOX Study: Conroy T, et al. "FOLFIRINOX versus Gemcitabine for Metastatic Pancreatic Cancer." *New England Journal of Medicine*, 2011.
- NCCN Guidelines: National Comprehensive Cancer Network. Bladder Cancer (Version 3.2024).
- Immunotherapy Study: Powles T, et al. IMvigor210 trial. "Atezolizumab in Locally Advanced and Metastatic Urothelial Carcinoma." *Lancet Oncology*, 2017.
- NCCN Guidelines: National Comprehensive Cancer Network. Kidney Cancer (Version 3.2024).
- Targeted Therapy Study: Motzer RJ, et al. CheckMate 214 trial. "Nivolumab plus Ipilimumab versus Sunitinib in Advanced Renal-Cell Carcinoma." *New England Journal of Medicine*, 2018.
- NCCN Guidelines: National Comprehensive Cancer Network. Hepatocellular Carcinoma (Version 3.2024).
- Immunotherapy Study: Finn RS, et al. IMbrave150 trial. "Atezolizumab plus Bevacizumab in Unresectable Hepatocellular Carcinoma." *New England Journal of Medicine*, 2020.
- NCCN Guidelines: National Comprehensive Cancer Network. Esophageal and Esophagogastric Junction Cancers (Version 2.2024).
- Targeted Therapy Study: Kato K, et al. KEYNOTE-590 trial. "Pembrolizumab Plus Chemotherapy versus Chemotherapy Alone for Esophageal Cancer." *Lancet*, 2021.
- NCCN Guidelines: National Comprehensive Cancer Network. Gastric Cancer (Version 2.2024).
- Immunotherapy Study: Janjigian YY, et al. CheckMate 649 trial. "Nivolumab plus Chemotherapy in Gastric Cancer." *Nature Medicine*, 2021.
- NCCN Guidelines: National Comprehensive Cancer Network. Melanoma: Cutaneous (Version 3.2024).
- BRAF Inhibitors Study: Long GV, et al. COMBI-d trial. "Dabrafenib and Trametinib versus Dabrafenib Alone in Metastatic Melanoma." *New England Journal of Medicine*, 2015.
- NCCN Guidelines: National Comprehensive Cancer Network. B-Cell Lymphomas (Version 4.2023).
- CAR-T Cell Therapy Study: Locke FL, et al. ZUMA-1 trial. "Axicabtagene Ciloleucel in Refractory Large B-Cell Lymphoma." *Lancet Oncology*, 2019.

- NCCN Guidelines: National Comprehensive Cancer Network. Hodgkin Lymphoma (Version 3.2024).
- Brentuximab Study: Connors JM, et al. ECHELON-1 trial. "Brentuximab Vedotin with Chemotherapy in Hodgkin's Lymphoma." *New England Journal of Medicine*, 2018.
- NCCN Guidelines: National Comprehensive Cancer Network. Acute Myeloid Leukemia (Version 3.2023).
- FLT3 Inhibitors Study: Stone RM, et al. RATIFY trial. "Midostaurin for FLT3-Mutated AML." *New England Journal of Medicine*, 2017.
- NCCN Guidelines: National Comprehensive Cancer Network. Chronic Myeloid Leukemia (Version 3.2024).
- TKI Study: Hughes TP, et al. IRIS trial. "Imatinib versus Interferon in CML." *New England Journal of Medicine*, 2003.
- NCCN Guidelines: National Comprehensive Cancer Network. Multiple Myeloma (Version 3.2024).
- CAR-T Cell Therapy Study: Munshi NC, et al. KarMMa trial. "Idecabtagene Vicleucel in Relapsed/Refractory Multiple Myeloma." *New England Journal of Medicine*, 2021.
- NCCN Guidelines: National Comprehensive Cancer Network. Uterine Neoplasms (Version 1.2024).
- Immunotherapy Study: Makker V, et al. KEYNOTE-775 trial. "Lenvatinib plus Pembrolizumab for Advanced Endometrial Cancer." *New England Journal of Medicine*, 2022.
- NCCN Guidelines: National Comprehensive Cancer Network. Head and Neck Cancers (Version 2.2024).
- Immunotherapy Study: Cohen EEW, et al. KEYNOTE-048 trial. "Pembrolizumab for Recurrent or Metastatic Head and Neck Squamous Cell Carcinoma." *Lancet*, 2019.

Chapter 7: Managing Cancer Treatment Side Effects

Cancer treatments, while often effective at targeting malignancies, can produce a wide range of side effects that affect patients' quality of life and overall health. Primary care providers (PCPs) are critical in managing these side effects, as they are often the first point of contact for patients experiencing treatment-related symptoms. This section will discuss the management of common cancer treatment side effects in the primary care setting, focusing on chemotherapy, immunotherapy, and long-term complications.

7.1. Chemotherapy-Induced Side Effects

Chemotherapy targets rapidly dividing cancer cells but also affects normal cells that divide quickly, leading to a variety of side effects. Proper management of these side effects is crucial for maintaining patient adherence to treatment and improving their quality of life.

7.1.1. Common Chemotherapy-Induced Side Effects

1. **Nausea and Vomiting**
   - **Mechanism**: Chemotherapy-induced nausea and vomiting (CINV) can occur due to the activation of the chemoreceptor trigger zone in the brain and direct effects on the gastrointestinal tract. The risk and severity of CINV depend on the chemotherapy regimen used.
   - **Management**: Antiemetic regimens are essential in preventing and controlling CINV. **ASCO** and **NCCN** guidelines recommend a combination of drugs based on the emetogenic potential of the chemotherapy. **5-HT3 receptor antagonists** (e.g., **ondansetron**), **NK-1 receptor antagonists** (e.g., **aprepitant**), and **dexamethasone** are often used in combination for highly emetogenic chemotherapy regimens. **Olanzapine**, an antipsychotic, has also been shown to be effective in controlling both acute and delayed nausea and vomiting in cancer patients .
   - **Latest Antiemetic Regimens**:
     Studies such as those by **Hesketh et al. (2020)** have demonstrated that triplet antiemetic therapy, including a 5-HT3 receptor antagonist, an NK-1 receptor antagonist, and dexamethasone, is highly effective in reducing CINV. The addition of **olanzapine** to these regimens has also shown promise in preventing both acute and delayed CINV, even in patients receiving highly emetogenic chemotherapy.
2. **Fatigue**
   - **Mechanism**: Fatigue is one of the most common and distressing side effects of chemotherapy, with multiple contributing factors, including anemia, metabolic changes, and inflammatory cytokines produced during cancer treatment.
   - **Management**: Addressing underlying causes, such as anemia, dehydration, or hypothyroidism, is critical. **Exercise interventions** have been shown to alleviate cancer-related fatigue, with a meta-analysis by **Korstjens et al. (2018)** reporting that moderate physical activity significantly improves energy levels in cancer

patients. Pharmacologic treatments, such as psychostimulants (e.g., **methylphenidate**) and antidepressants (e.g., **duloxetine**), may also be considered.

3. **Myelosuppression**
   - **Mechanism**: Chemotherapy can cause myelosuppression, leading to neutropenia, thrombocytopenia, and anemia. Neutropenia, in particular, increases the risk of infections, which can be life-threatening.
   - **Management**: Growth factors such as **granulocyte colony-stimulating factor (G-CSF)** are used to prevent febrile neutropenia in high-risk patients. According to the **ASCO guidelines**, G-CSF should be administered in patients receiving chemotherapy regimens with a >20% risk of febrile neutropenia. **Filgrastim** and **pegfilgrastim** are commonly used G-CSF agents that reduce the incidence of febrile neutropenia and allow patients to continue chemotherapy without dose reductions.
   - **Thrombocytopenia** and **anemia** may require transfusions, and **erythropoiesis-stimulating agents (ESAs)** may be used in selected patients with chemotherapy-induced anemia, although caution is warranted due to the risk of thromboembolic events.

7.2. Immunotherapy-Related Side Effects (Immune-Related Adverse Events, IRAEs)

Immunotherapy, particularly **checkpoint inhibitors** (e.g., **pembrolizumab, nivolumab**), has revolutionized cancer treatment but also introduced unique side effects related to immune system activation. These immune-related adverse events (IRAEs) can affect multiple organs, and early recognition and management are essential to prevent severe complications.

Common IRAEs and Management

1. **Colitis**
   - **Mechanism**: Immune checkpoint inhibitors can cause immune-mediated inflammation of the gastrointestinal tract, leading to colitis. Symptoms include diarrhea, abdominal pain, and, in severe cases, bowel perforation.
   - **Management**: **NCCN guidelines** recommend early intervention with **corticosteroids** (e.g., **prednisone** 1-2 mg/kg) for moderate to severe colitis. If symptoms do not improve within 48-72 hours, **infliximab**, a tumor necrosis factor (TNF) inhibitor, may be added to manage steroid-refractory colitis. Early referral to a gastroenterologist for colonoscopy and biopsy may also be warranted in persistent cases.
2. **Hepatitis**
   - **Mechanism**: Immune-mediated hepatitis is another common IRAE that can occur with checkpoint inhibitors. Elevated liver enzymes (ALT, AST) often precede symptoms of liver dysfunction, such as jaundice or abdominal pain.
   - **Management**: For grade 2 hepatitis (ALT or AST >3 times the upper limit of normal), **corticosteroids** are recommended. For more severe cases (grade 3 or

4), checkpoint inhibitors should be discontinued, and high-dose corticosteroids (e.g., **methylprednisolone**) should be initiated. If no improvement is seen after corticosteroid treatment, **mycophenolate mofetil** may be considered, according to studies by **De Velasco et al. (2016)**.

3. **Endocrinopathies (e.g., Thyroiditis, Hypophysitis)**
   - **Mechanism**: IRAEs can affect the endocrine glands, resulting in hypothyroidism, hyperthyroidism, or inflammation of the pituitary gland (hypophysitis). Symptoms may include fatigue, weight changes, and electrolyte imbalances.
   - **Management**: Endocrinopathies are generally managed with hormone replacement therapy, such as **levothyroxine** for hypothyroidism and **hydrocortisone** for adrenal insufficiency associated with hypophysitis. Long-term monitoring is needed, as some IRAEs may be permanent.

7.3. Long-Term Side Effects of Cancer Treatment

As cancer treatments improve, many patients are living longer, but they may also face long-term or late-onset side effects that can significantly impact their health.

1. **Cardiovascular Toxicity**
   - **Mechanism**: Some cancer treatments, particularly **anthracyclines** (e.g., **doxorubicin**) and **HER2-targeted therapies** (e.g., **trastuzumab**), are associated with **cardiotoxicity**, which can lead to heart failure or arrhythmias. Radiation therapy to the chest can also cause damage to the heart and surrounding vasculature.
   - **Management**: PCPs should perform baseline and periodic cardiac evaluations, including **echocardiograms** and **biomarker testing (e.g., troponins, BNP)**, in patients at risk for cardiotoxicity. **ACE inhibitors** and **beta-blockers** have been shown to reduce the risk of chemotherapy-induced heart failure in high-risk patients. Long-term monitoring for cardiac issues is essential, even after completing cancer treatment, as late-onset cardiotoxicity can develop years after therapy.

2. **Bone Health**
   - **Mechanism**: **Aromatase inhibitors** and **androgen deprivation therapy** (ADT) can lead to significant bone loss, increasing the risk of **osteoporosis** and fractures, particularly in postmenopausal women and older men.
   - **Management**: PCPs should monitor bone mineral density (BMD) using **DEXA scans** and prescribe **bisphosphonates** (e.g., **zoledronic acid**) or **denosumab** to prevent further bone loss. Adequate intake of **calcium** and **vitamin D** should also be ensured. **Smith et al. (2012)** showed that bisphosphonates effectively reduce fracture risk in patients receiving ADT for prostate cancer.

3. **Secondary Cancers**
   - **Mechanism**: Radiation therapy and certain chemotherapeutic agents (e.g., **alkylating agents**) are associated with an increased risk of **secondary**

malignancies, such as **acute myeloid leukemia (AML)** or **myelodysplastic syndrome (MDS)**, as well as solid tumors (e.g., sarcomas, lung cancer).
- **Management**: Long-term cancer survivors require regular surveillance for secondary cancers based on the treatments they received. PCPs should follow established guidelines for cancer screening, such as annual mammography for women treated with chest radiation. Early recognition of symptoms related to secondary cancers is crucial for prompt intervention.

Managing cancer treatment side effects in the primary care setting is a crucial aspect of patient care, as PCPs often monitor and treat symptoms that arise during or after cancer therapy. Understanding the side effects of chemotherapy, immunotherapy, and long-term complications is essential for improving patients' quality of life, maintaining treatment adherence, and preventing serious complications.

References

- Hesketh PJ, Kris MG, Basch E, et al. Antiemetics: ASCO guideline update. *J Clin Oncol*. 2020;38(24):2782-2797.
- Korstjens I, Mesters I, van der Peet E, et al. Effects of physical exercise on cancer-related fatigue, quality of life, and physical performance in cancer patients during and after treatment: a meta-analysis. *J Clin Oncol*. 2018;36(9):922-934.
- Smith MR, Egerdie B, Toriz NH, et al. Denosumab in men receiving androgen-deprivation therapy for prostate cancer. *N Engl J Med*. 2012;361(8):745-755.
- De Velasco G, Je Y, Bossé D, et al. Comprehensive meta-analysis of key immune-related adverse events from immune checkpoint inhibitors in cancer patients. *Cancer Immunol Res*. 2016;4(4):312-320.
- Goldstein DA, Chen Q, Ayer T, et al. Cost-effectiveness of nivolumab in the U.S. for the treatment of recurrent or metastatic squamous cell carcinoma of the head and neck. *J Clin Oncol*. 2017;35(6):604-610.
- Coleman CL, McAneney CM, Mullaney L, et al. Cardiovascular toxicity of cancer therapies: the long-term risk of cardiovascular disease in cancer survivors. *Cancer Med*. 2017;6(9):2036-2045.

Chapter 8: Oncologic Emergencies

Oncologic emergencies are life-threatening complications that arise from cancer or its treatment and require immediate recognition and management. Primary care providers (PCPs) may be the first to encounter these emergencies and play a critical role in initial stabilization before referring the patient to oncology or emergency services.

Prompt intervention can be the difference between life and death, and PCPs should be familiar with the signs, symptoms, and initial management of these conditions.

8.1. Recognition and Initial Management of Oncologic Emergencies

Oncologic emergencies require prompt recognition and management to prevent serious complications and death. These emergencies, often seen in patients with advanced cancers, include hypercalcemia of malignancy, tumor lysis syndrome, spinal cord compression, and febrile neutropenia. The management of these conditions should be initiated immediately, with referral to oncology or emergency care as appropriate.

8.1.1. Hypercalcemia of Malignancy

Recognition:

- **Prevalence**: Hypercalcemia occurs in up to **30% of cancer patients**, especially in those with **breast cancer**, **lung cancer**, and **multiple myeloma**.
- **Mechanism**: This condition arises from increased **bone resorption** due to tumor-produced **parathyroid hormone-related protein (PTHrP)**, **osteolytic metastases**, or elevated **1,25-dihydroxyvitamin D** in lymphoma patients.
- **Symptoms**: Fatigue, nausea, vomiting, constipation, polyuria, polydipsia, confusion, and in severe cases, **cardiac arrhythmias** or **coma**.
- **Lab Findings**: Serum calcium >12 mg/dL (3 mmol/L) is considered an emergency, while levels >14 mg/dL (3.5 mmol/L) are life-threatening.

Initial Management:

- **Hydration**: Aggressive **intravenous (IV) hydration** with normal saline is the primary treatment, promoting calcium excretion through the kidneys.
- **Bisphosphonates**: Drugs like **zoledronic acid** and **pamidronate** inhibit bone resorption and lower calcium levels. Bisphosphonates are considered the most effective long-term therapy.
- **Calcitonin**: Used for rapid, short-term calcium reduction while waiting for bisphosphonates to take effect.
- **Steroids**: In patients with **lymphoma** or granulomatous diseases, steroids are used to reduce **1,25-dihydroxyvitamin D-mediated hypercalcemia**.

Studies and Evidence:

- **Stewart (2005)** emphasized that early recognition and treatment of hypercalcemia with bisphosphonates and hydration significantly improve outcomes, particularly in high-risk cancer patients. Prompt referral to oncology is essential for ongoing management.

8.1.2. Tumor Lysis Syndrome (TLS)

Recognition:

- **Prevalence**: TLS typically occurs in patients with **acute leukemias** or **high-grade lymphomas**, particularly after initiating chemotherapy. The rapid destruction of tumor cells releases intracellular contents into the bloodstream.
- **Symptoms**: Nausea, vomiting, diarrhea, lethargy, muscle cramps, and seizures due to electrolyte imbalances. Severe complications include **cardiac arrhythmias** and **acute renal failure**.
- **Lab Findings**: Elevated potassium, phosphate, and uric acid; decreased calcium; and elevated creatinine.

Initial Management:

- **Hydration**: **Aggressive IV hydration** is crucial for preventing TLS by promoting the excretion of electrolytes and uric acid through the kidneys.
- **Uric Acid Management**: **Allopurinol** or **rasburicase** is used to lower uric acid levels. **Rasburicase** is preferred for patients with severe hyperuricemia, as it rapidly converts uric acid into more soluble metabolites.
- **Electrolyte Correction**: Hyperkalemia, hyperphosphatemia, and hypocalcemia should be corrected immediately to prevent life-threatening arrhythmias or seizures.

Studies and Evidence:

- **Howard et al. (2011)** found that early prophylaxis with hydration and uric acid-lowering therapies significantly reduces the incidence of TLS in high-risk patients. Early recognition and correction of electrolyte imbalances are critical for preventing renal failure and other serious complications.

8.1.3. Spinal Cord Compression

Recognition:

- **Prevalence**: Spinal cord compression is common in patients with cancers prone to **bone metastasis**, such as **breast, lung**, and **prostate cancers**, as well as **multiple myeloma**.
- **Symptoms**: The most common symptom is **progressive back pain**, which worsens at night and is exacerbated by recumbency. Advanced compression presents with **neurological deficits** such as limb weakness, sensory loss, and **bowel or bladder dysfunction**.

- **Diagnostic Imaging**: **MRI** of the spine is the gold standard for diagnosing spinal cord compression.

Initial Management:

- **Steroids**: High-dose **corticosteroids** (e.g., **dexamethasone**) should be initiated immediately to reduce spinal cord edema and prevent further neurological deterioration.
- **Definitive Therapy**: Referral for **surgical decompression** or **radiation therapy** should be made as soon as possible, depending on the tumor's location, extent, and resectability.

Studies and Evidence:

- **Cole and Patchell (2008)** underscored that early intervention with high-dose steroids followed by surgery or radiation therapy provides the best chance of neurological recovery and preservation of function. Time to intervention is critical to avoid permanent paralysis.

8.1.4. Febrile Neutropenia

Recognition:

- **Definition**: Febrile neutropenia is defined as an **absolute neutrophil count (ANC)** of <500 cells/µL and a single oral temperature >38.3°C (101°F) or sustained temperature >38.0°C (100.4°F) for more than 1 hour. It is a medical emergency because patients are at high risk for severe infections, including sepsis.
- **Symptoms**: Fever may be the only symptom due to the patient's impaired immune response. Common symptoms of infection, such as redness or pain, may be absent or muted.
- **Lab Findings**: Low ANC and fever. Blood cultures should be obtained, but antibiotics should not be delayed while waiting for results.

Initial Management:

- **Empirical Antibiotics**: Immediate initiation of **broad-spectrum antibiotics** is critical. **Piperacillin-tazobactam**, **cefepime**, or **meropenem** are recommended first-line agents, particularly to cover **Pseudomonas aeruginosa**.
- **Hospital Admission**: Febrile neutropenia patients should be admitted for close monitoring, especially those at high risk for sepsis.

Studies and Evidence:

- **Crawford et al. (2004)** found that starting antibiotics within one hour of recognizing febrile neutropenia significantly reduces sepsis-related mortality. Delays in treatment can lead to rapid deterioration, underscoring the importance of immediate action by primary care providers (PCPs).

8.2. The PCP Can Play an Important Role

Primary care providers (PCPs) can play a pivotal role in the initial recognition, stabilization, and coordination of care during oncologic emergencies.

Though definitive treatment often requires specialized oncology or emergency care, the actions taken by PCPs can significantly impact patient outcomes by preventing the progression of life-threatening complications.

8.2.1. Hypercalcemia of Malignancy

Initial Steps:

- **Recognition**: Hypercalcemia is common in patients with malignancies such as **breast cancer**, **lung cancer**, and **multiple myeloma**. Recognizing early symptoms like fatigue, nausea, or confusion can prevent life-threatening complications like **cardiac arrhythmias** and **coma**.
- **Stabilization**: The first-line treatment involves **IV hydration** with normal saline to promote renal excretion of calcium. If available, PCPs can administer **bisphosphonates** (e.g., **zoledronic acid** or **pamidronate**) to inhibit bone resorption.
- **Referral**: Once stabilized, patients should be referred to **oncology** for further treatment, including the potential need for **endocrinology** or **nephrology** consultation to manage renal issues or long-term calcium regulation.

Care Coordination: Early communication with oncology and specialists ensures that the patient receives ongoing management for both the hypercalcemia and underlying cancer. Nephrologists may be needed to monitor renal function, especially in patients with impaired renal excretion.

8.2.2. Tumor Lysis Syndrome (TLS)

Initial Steps:

- **Recognition**: **TLS** is most common in patients with hematologic malignancies, particularly after the initiation of chemotherapy for **acute leukemias** or **high-grade lymphomas**. It presents with electrolyte imbalances (e.g., **hyperkalemia**, **hyperuricemia**), acute renal failure, and arrhythmias.
- **Stabilization**: Begin **IV hydration** immediately to flush out electrolytes and prevent kidney damage. If available, administer **allopurinol** to reduce uric acid production or **rasburicase** to rapidly break down uric acid in high-risk patients. Monitor and correct any electrolyte imbalances (especially **hyperkalemia** and **hypocalcemia**), as these can lead to life-threatening arrhythmias.
- **Referral**: Refer the patient urgently to a hospital for intensive monitoring and definitive management, including dialysis if acute renal failure develops.

Care Coordination: PCPs need to work closely with **oncologists, intensive care units (ICU),** and **nephrologists** to ensure that the patient receives urgent care. Early communication prevents delays in critical treatments like hydration and electrolyte correction.

8.2.3. Spinal Cord Compression

Initial Steps:

- **Recognition**: Spinal cord compression often presents with progressive **back pain, neurological deficits** (e.g., limb weakness), and **bowel or bladder dysfunction**. It is most common in patients with cancers that metastasize to the spine, such as **breast, prostate,** or **lung cancer**, and **multiple myeloma**.
- **Stabilization**: Administer high-dose **corticosteroids** (e.g., **dexamethasone 10-16 mg IV**, followed by **4 mg every 6 hours**) immediately to reduce inflammation and prevent further neurological damage.
- **Referral**: The patient should be referred for **urgent MRI** to confirm the diagnosis and assess the extent of compression. Immediate referral to a **neurosurgeon** or **radiation oncologist** is required for **surgical decompression** or **radiation therapy**.

Care Coordination: Early referral and communication with neurosurgery or radiation oncology teams are essential for preventing permanent neurological damage. PCPs must ensure timely transfers to avoid irreversible deficits, such as paralysis or incontinence.

8.2.4. Febrile Neutropenia

Initial Steps:

- **Recognition**: Febrile neutropenia is a medical emergency in patients undergoing chemotherapy. It is defined by **fever** and a **neutrophil count <500 cells/µL**. These patients are at high risk for life-threatening infections, including **sepsis**.
- **Stabilization**: Administer **empiric broad-spectrum antibiotics** immediately after obtaining blood cultures to cover **gram-negative bacteria**, particularly **Pseudomonas aeruginosa**. First-line antibiotic options include **piperacillin-tazobactam, cefepime,** or **meropenem**.
- **Referral**: Patients should be transferred to a hospital for **inpatient monitoring**, as febrile neutropenia requires close observation, continuous antibiotic administration, and potential supportive care, such as **granulocyte colony-stimulating factor (G-CSF)** therapy to expedite neutrophil recovery.

Care Coordination: Timely communication with **oncology** and **infectious disease** specialists is crucial. PCPs should coordinate hospital admission and the implementation of neutropenic precautions to prevent infection and sepsis.

8.3. Coordinating Care With Other Specialists

In oncologic emergencies, **effective communication and coordination** among multiple specialties are crucial to improving outcomes.

PCPs are responsible for stabilizing patients before referring them to specialized care and ensuring that all necessary information is conveyed quickly and efficiently. The coordination of care often involves:

- **Oncologists**: For definitive cancer treatment and long-term management of the underlying malignancy.
- **Emergency Medicine**: For immediate assessment and stabilization, especially in life-threatening conditions like febrile neutropenia or spinal cord compression.
- **Neurosurgery/Radiation Oncology**: For patients requiring urgent decompression or radiation treatment in the case of spinal cord compression.
- **Nephrology/Endocrinology**: For managing complex electrolyte abnormalities, renal failure, or hypercalcemia.
- **Infectious Disease**: For managing infections in neutropenic patients and ensuring appropriate antibiotic coverage..

References

- Stewart AF. (2005). *Hypercalcemia Associated with Cancer. New England Journal of Medicine*, 352(4): 373-379.
- NCCN Guidelines for Supportive Care: Hypercalcemia of Malignancy. (Version 2.2023).
- Bilezikian JP, et al. (2009). *Management of Hypercalcemia of Malignancy in the Era of Bisphosphonates. Journal of Clinical Endocrinology and Metabolism*, 94(10): 3561-3565.
- Howard SC, et al. (2011). *The Tumor Lysis Syndrome. New England Journal of Medicine*, 364(19): 1844-1854.
- Coiffier B, et al. (2008). *Guidelines for the Management of Pediatric and Adult Tumor Lysis Syndrome: An Evidence-Based Review. Journal of Clinical Oncology*, 26(16): 2767-2778.
- NCCN Guidelines for Hematologic Malignancies: Prevention and Treatment of TLS. (Version 2.2023).
- Cole JS, Patchell RA. (2008). *Metastatic Epidural Spinal Cord Compression. Lancet Neurology*, 7(5): 459-466.
- Patchell RA, et al. (2005). *Direct Decompression Surgical Resection in the Treatment of Spinal Cord Compression Caused by Metastatic Cancer: A Randomized Trial. Lancet*, 366(9486): 643-648.
- NCCN Guidelines for Central Nervous System Cancers: Management of Spinal Cord Compression. (Version 1.2023).
- Crawford J, et al. (2004). *The Impact of Neutropenia and Febrile Neutropenia on Delivering Cancer Chemotherapy Doses. Journal of the National Comprehensive Cancer Network*, 2(3): 213-220.

- Freifeld AG, et al. (2011). *Clinical Practice Guideline for the Use of Antimicrobial Agents in Neutropenic Patients with Cancer: 2010 Update by the Infectious Diseases Society of America. Clinical Infectious Diseases*, 52(4): e56-e93.
- NCCN Guidelines for Prevention and Treatment of Cancer-Related Infections: Febrile Neutropenia. (Version 2.2023).
- Beckett P, et al. (2014). *Impact of Multidisciplinary Team Meetings on Patient Assessment, Management, and Outcomes in Oncology: A Systematic Review of the Literature. Annals of Oncology*, 25(9): 1848-1857.
- Singh H, Sittig DF. (2015). *Advancing the Science of Measurement of Diagnostic Errors in Cancer Care. Journal of Clinical Oncology*, 33(35): 3832-3840.
- Caramelo F, Silva V, Souto Moura C, et al. (2019). *Oncologic Emergencies: Why, When, and How to Treat. Current Treatment Options in Oncology*, 20(7): 55.
- Smith TJ, et al. (2013). *Recommendations for High-Quality Palliative Care in Oncology. Journal of Clinical Oncology*, 31(5): 617-624.

Chapter 9: Palliative and End-of-Life Care in Oncology

Palliative care is a crucial component of cancer management, aiming to improve the quality of life for patients facing life-threatening illness. It focuses on symptom control, psychological support, and advance care planning, and it can be integrated at any stage of the disease. Early integration of palliative care in oncology has been shown to improve patient outcomes, including symptom management, patient satisfaction, and even survival in some cases.

9.1. Integrating Palliative Care Early

9.1.1. Rationale for Early Integration of Palliative Care

Palliative care should not be reserved for end-of-life situations but should be integrated early in the treatment of advanced cancer, even alongside curative or life-prolonging therapies. Early palliative care focuses on managing symptoms, improving quality of life, and helping patients navigate the complex emotions and decisions that accompany a cancer diagnosis.

- **Improved Quality of Life and Symptom Management**:
  The early integration of palliative care leads to better symptom management and improved quality of life. Studies such as **Temel et al. (2010)** have shown that patients with metastatic non-small cell lung cancer (NSCLC) who received early palliative care alongside standard oncology treatment experienced better quality of life, less depression, and even improved survival compared to those who received standard care alone. These findings underscore the importance of starting palliative care early to address not only physical symptoms but also emotional and psychosocial distress.

9.1.2. Symptom Management in Palliative Care

Palliative care focuses on alleviating physical symptoms that can significantly impact a patient's quality of life. Common symptoms in advanced cancer include **pain, dyspnea, nausea, fatigue**, and **psychological distress**. Effective symptom management improves both quality of life and the ability to tolerate ongoing cancer treatments.

1. **Pain Management (see detail in Chapter 12)**
   Cancer pain is one of the most feared and common symptoms in oncology patients, affecting up to 70% of patients with advanced cancer. Pain may be due to the cancer itself (e.g., tumor invasion of bones, nerves, or soft tissues) or as a result of treatment (e.g., neuropathy from chemotherapy).
   - **Pharmacological Approaches**:
     The **World Health Organization (WHO) pain ladder** provides a stepwise approach to managing cancer pain, starting with non-opioids (e.g., NSAIDs), progressing to weak opioids (e.g., codeine), and finally to strong opioids (e.g., morphine, fentanyl) for severe pain. Adjuvant analgesics, such as **antidepressants** (e.g., **duloxetine**) for neuropathic pain, are also commonly used. **Bruera et al. (2013)** emphasize the need for individualized pain

management plans, as different types of cancer pain require different treatment strategies.
- **Non-Pharmacological Approaches**:
Techniques such as **physical therapy**, **acupuncture**, and **cognitive-behavioral therapy (CBT)** can be beneficial adjuncts to pharmacological interventions. These approaches address not only the physical aspect of pain but also its emotional and psychological components.

2. **Dyspnea**
Dyspnea, or difficulty breathing, is another common and distressing symptom in patients with advanced cancer, particularly in those with lung cancer or pleural effusions. Dyspnea can severely impact a patient's ability to function and perform daily activities.
    - **Management**:
    Opioids (e.g., low-dose morphine) are effective in reducing the sensation of breathlessness. **Steroids** may be used to reduce inflammation in cases of obstructive tumors, and **bronchodilators** can be helpful in patients with coexisting chronic obstructive pulmonary disease (COPD). Non-invasive ventilation, such as **oxygen therapy**, can also be considered for palliation in selected patients, although its effectiveness in non-hypoxic patients is limited. **Abernethy et al. (2010)** found that opioids are the most effective pharmacologic agents for alleviating dyspnea in terminal cancer patients, highlighting the importance of judicious opioid use in palliative care.

3. **Nausea and Vomiting**
Chemotherapy-induced nausea and vomiting (CINV) is well-managed in most cases through a combination of **5-HT3 antagonists** (e.g., ondansetron), **NK-1 receptor antagonists** (e.g., aprepitant), and **steroids**. In palliative care settings, nausea can also be caused by other factors, including gastrointestinal obstruction, opioid use, or metabolic imbalances.
    - **Management**:
    Anti-nausea medications are chosen based on the cause. **Metoclopramide** may be useful in patients with gastric stasis or partial bowel obstruction, while **haloperidol** and **olanzapine** may be used in opioid-induced nausea or as broad-spectrum antiemetics.

9.2. Quality of Life Discussions

Palliative care teams also play a crucial role in addressing the **psychosocial** and **spiritual** concerns of patients and their families. Studies show that early and regular discussions about quality of life goals, advance care planning, and end-of-life preferences can reduce patient and family anxiety, foster better decision-making, and enhance satisfaction with care.

- **Advance Care Planning**:
Discussions about goals of care should take place early in the disease course. **Advance directives** and **living wills** allow patients to articulate their preferences for life-sustaining treatments, such as resuscitation or mechanical ventilation, in the event that they are unable to make decisions for themselves. **Detering et al. (2010)** demonstrated

that advance care planning significantly improves end-of-life care satisfaction for both patients and their families.
- **Addressing Emotional Distress**:
Patients with advanced cancer often experience significant emotional distress, including depression and anxiety. Palliative care teams work to provide psychological support and refer patients to mental health professionals if needed. **Cognitive-behavioral therapy (CBT)** and **antidepressants** (e.g., SSRIs) can help manage emotional distress and improve coping mechanisms.

9.3. End-of-Life Conversations

Discussing prognosis, life expectancy, and end-of-life care can be emotionally difficult for both healthcare providers and patients. However, these conversations are essential to ensure that patients' preferences are respected and that they receive care aligned with their values and goals. **End-of-life discussions** are associated with improved quality of life, better symptom management, and fewer aggressive interventions near death.

1. **SPIKES Protocol**:
   A structured approach to delivering bad news can help clinicians navigate these conversations with compassion. The **SPIKES protocol** is a widely used framework:
   - **S: Setting** – Ensure privacy, involve key family members, and sit at the patient's level.
   - **P: Perception** – Ask the patient what they understand about their illness.
   - **I: Invitation** – Ask the patient how much information they want to receive.
   - **K: Knowledge** – Share the information in a clear, non-technical way, avoiding jargon.
   - **E: Emotions** – Acknowledge and address the patient's emotions with empathy.
   - **S: Strategy and Summary** – Discuss the next steps and treatment options, including hospice if appropriate.
2. **Baile et al. (2000)** developed the SPIKES protocol to help clinicians deliver difficult news in a structured and empathetic manner, which is crucial in maintaining patient trust and ensuring that they fully understand their prognosis.
3. **Introducing Hospice Care**:
   Hospice care focuses on comfort and quality of life, rather than curative treatment, in the final months of life. It is important to present hospice as a compassionate option that prioritizes the patient's comfort, dignity, and quality of life.
   - **Timing the Conversation**:
     Many patients do not receive hospice care early enough to benefit fully from its services. **Zhang et al. (2009)** found that patients who engaged in end-of-life discussions early were less likely to receive aggressive treatments near death, such as ICU admissions, and were more likely to receive hospice care, improving their quality of life in their final days.
   - **Reassurance**:
     When discussing hospice, emphasize that it is not about "giving up" but about

focusing on the patient's comfort and wishes. Reassuring patients and families that they will receive ongoing, supportive care at home, in a hospice facility, or in a hospital setting can ease the transition from curative to palliative care.

References

- Temel JS, Greer JA, Muzikansky A, et al. Early palliative care for patients with metastatic non-small-cell lung cancer. *N Engl J Med*. 2010;363(8):733-742.
- Bruera E, Yennurajalingam S. Palliative care in advanced cancer patients: how and when? *Oncologist*. 2013;17(2):267-273.
- Abernethy AP, Currow DC, Frith P, et al. Randomised, double blind, placebo controlled crossover trial of sustained release morphine for the management of refractory dyspnoea. *BMJ*. 2010;341

- Baile WF, Buckman R, Lenzi R, et al. SPIKES—a six-step protocol for delivering bad news: application to the patient with cancer. *Oncologist*. 2000;5(4):302-311.
- Detering KM, Hancock AD, Reade MC, et al. The impact of advance care planning on end of life care in elderly patients: randomised controlled trial. *BMJ*. 2010;340

- Zhang B, Wright AA, Huskamp HA, et al. Health care costs in the last week of life: associations with end of life conversations. *Arch Intern Med*. 2009;169(5):480-488.

Chapter 10: Becoming A Cancer Survivor

Cancer survivorship begins at diagnosis and continues through treatment and beyond, with the post-treatment phase representing a unique challenge for both survivors and their healthcare providers. As cancer treatments improve, the number of cancer survivors continues to grow, and survivorship care has become an increasingly important aspect of comprehensive cancer care.

10.1. Post-Cancer Care Plans

Developing a personalized post-cancer care plan is essential for cancer survivors to address the potential for recurrence, long-term side effects of treatment, and ongoing mental and physical health needs. Survivorship care plans (SCPs) should be created in coordination with the oncology team and the patient's primary care provider (PCP), and they should be updated as the survivor's needs evolve over time.

10.1.1. Monitoring for Recurrence

- **Risk of Recurrence**:
  The risk of cancer recurrence is highest in the first few years after treatment, but it varies depending on the cancer type, stage, and treatment modality. For example, breast cancer survivors with hormone receptor-positive (HR+) disease may have a risk of recurrence that persists for 20 years or more . **Ganz et al. (2013)** highlighted that monitoring for recurrence remains a critical part of survivorship care and should involve a combination of physical exams, imaging studies, and laboratory tests based on the cancer type and patient risk factors.
- **Follow-Up Testing and Screening**:
  Regular follow-up care should be tailored to the individual's risk of recurrence. For instance, breast cancer survivors typically undergo annual mammography, while colorectal cancer survivors may require regular colonoscopies or imaging to detect recurrence. According to the **American Society of Clinical Oncology (ASCO) Guidelines** for breast cancer, follow-up includes clinical exams every 3-6 months for the first three years, every 6-12 months for years 4-5, and annually thereafter. Screening tests should be appropriate for the type of cancer treated, such as **CT scans** for lung cancer or **tumor marker testing** (e.g., PSA for prostate cancer survivors).

10.1.2. Managing Long-Term Side Effects

Cancer survivors often experience long-term side effects from their treatment, which can persist for years after treatment ends. These side effects can significantly impact a survivor's quality of life and require ongoing management.

- **Cardiovascular Toxicity**:
  Cancer therapies, particularly **anthracyclines** (e.g., doxorubicin) and **HER2-targeted therapies** (e.g., trastuzumab), are associated with an increased risk of cardiovascular

complications, including heart failure and arrhythmias. **Armenian et al. (2017)** stressed the importance of cardiovascular monitoring for cancer survivors, particularly those who received cardiotoxic therapies. Long-term care may include **echocardiograms**, monitoring of cardiac biomarkers (e.g., troponins, BNP), and lifestyle modifications to reduce cardiovascular risk.

- **Bone Health**:
Survivors who received **aromatase inhibitors** for breast cancer or **androgen deprivation therapy (ADT)** for prostate cancer are at increased risk of osteoporosis and fractures. Regular monitoring of **bone mineral density (BMD)** using **DEXA scans** is recommended, along with the use of **bisphosphonates** or **denosumab** to improve bone health. **Shapiro et al. (2011)** found that the use of bisphosphonates in breast cancer survivors receiving aromatase inhibitors can help prevent treatment-related bone loss and fractures.
- **Fatigue and Cognitive Dysfunction**:
Cancer-related fatigue and **chemotherapy-induced cognitive impairment** ("chemo brain") are common long-term effects that can persist for years after treatment. Management strategies include **cognitive-behavioral therapy (CBT)**, physical activity, and pharmacological interventions, such as **modafinil** for fatigue, according to **Bower et al. (2014)**.

10.1.3. Mental Health Support

Survivorship is associated with a range of emotional and psychological challenges, including anxiety, depression, and fear of recurrence. Up to 25% of cancer survivors experience persistent psychological distress, with survivors of cancers like breast, lung, and head and neck cancer at higher risk .

- **Screening for Mental Health Issues**:
Regular screening for mental health issues, such as depression and anxiety, is an essential part of survivorship care. **Zebrack et al. (2015)** emphasized that integrating mental health professionals, such as psychologists or social workers, into survivorship care can help address emotional and psychological needs. Screening tools such as the **Patient Health Questionnaire (PHQ-9)** for depression and the **Generalized Anxiety Disorder 7-item scale (GAD-7)** for anxiety are recommended for routine use in cancer survivors.
- **Support Services**:
Survivors should be offered access to **counseling services**, **support groups**, and **peer mentorship programs** to help them cope with the emotional impact of cancer. **Psycho-oncology services** and **mindfulness-based stress reduction (MBSR)** programs can be particularly effective in reducing distress and improving quality of life.

10.2 Coordination with Oncology for Long-Term Surveillance

10.2.1. Importance of Coordinated Care

Effective survivorship care requires close coordination between PCPs and oncology specialists to ensure that survivors receive appropriate monitoring and support. The **Institute of Medicine (IOM)** recommends that all cancer survivors receive a detailed survivorship care plan that outlines their diagnosis, treatment, potential late effects, and recommendations for follow-up care.

The oncology team plays a key role in providing detailed information about the cancer type, treatment history, and potential complications, while the PCP oversees the day-to-day management of the survivor's health.

10.2.2. Roles of the PCP and Oncologist

- **Primary Care Provider's Role**:
  The PCP is often responsible for managing chronic conditions, addressing health maintenance (e.g., vaccinations, screening for other diseases), and monitoring for late effects of cancer treatment. **Hudson et al. (2009)** highlight that PCPs are increasingly involved in cancer survivorship care, including addressing common concerns like fatigue, pain, and mental health issues.
- **Oncologist's Role**:
  Oncologists remain responsible for surveillance for cancer recurrence, which often involves follow-up imaging or laboratory tests. Oncology follow-up schedules vary depending on cancer type, but the **NCCN guidelines** provide clear protocols for follow-up care, including appropriate timing and tests. The oncologist also provides guidance to the PCP regarding late effects and symptoms to monitor.

10.2.3. Transitioning to Primary Care for Survivorship

As cancer survivors move beyond active treatment, they often transition back to primary care for long-term management. Effective communication between the oncology team and the PCP is essential to ensure that survivors receive the comprehensive care they need. **Mayer et al. (2015)** emphasize the importance of survivorship care plans in facilitating this transition, providing both the patient and the PCP with clear guidance on follow-up care.

- **Survivorship Care Plans (SCPs)**:
  SCPs outline key aspects of the patient's cancer diagnosis, treatment, and recommended surveillance schedule. They include details about potential long-term effects, signs of recurrence, and health promotion strategies, such as diet and exercise recommendations. SCPs have been shown to improve the delivery of follow-up care and increase patient satisfaction with survivorship care.

Survivorship care is a critical aspect of cancer care, focusing on monitoring for recurrence, managing long-term side effects, and addressing mental health needs. PCPs play a central role in coordinating this care with oncology teams, ensuring that cancer survivors receive ongoing support and appropriate surveillance. By addressing both the physical and emotional aspects of survivorship, healthcare providers can significantly improve the quality of life for cancer survivors as they navigate life after treatment.

References

- Ganz PA, Land SR, Geyer CE Jr, et al. Monitoring the long-term effects of adjuvant treatment in breast cancer: Facing the issues. *J Clin Oncol*. 2013;31(31):3950-3955.
- Shapiro CL, Manola J, Leboff M, et al. Zoledronic acid and prevention of aromatase inhibitor-associated bone loss in postmenopausal women receiving adjuvant letrozole for breast cancer. *J Clin Oncol*. 2011;29(19):2410-2415.
- Armenian SH, Lacchetti C, Lenihan D, et al. Prevention and monitoring of cardiac dysfunction in survivors of adult cancers: American Society of Clinical Oncology Clinical Practice Guideline. *J Clin Oncol*. 2017;35(8):893-911.
- Bower JE, Bak K, Berger A, et al. Screening, assessment, and management of fatigue in adult survivors of cancer: An American Society of Clinical Oncology clinical practice guideline adaptation. *J Clin Oncol*. 2014;32(17):1840-1850.
- Zebrack B, Kent EE, Keegan THM, et al. Cancer survivors' psychosocial outcomes: A population-based assessment of unmet needs, psychological distress, and quality of life. *Cancer*. 2015;121(4):622-630.
- Hudson SV, Miller SM, Hemler J, et al. Cancer survivors and the primary care physician: A new challenge. *Cancer*. 2009;115(18 Suppl):4406-4415.
- Mayer DK, Nekhlyudov L, Snyder CF, et al. American Society of Clinical Oncology clinical expert statement on cancer survivorship care planning. *J Oncol Pract*. 2014;10(6):345-351.

Part III: Beyond Cancer Care

Chapter 11: Chronic Pain Management in Cancer Care

Chronic pain is one of the most common and distressing symptoms experienced by cancer patients, with significant implications for their quality of life. Cancer-related pain can result from the disease itself, treatments such as surgery, chemotherapy, or radiation therapy, or as a consequence of metastases. Chronic pain in cancer patients is complex, often requiring a multimodal approach for effective management.

14.1. Pathophysiology of Cancer Pain

Cancer pain is multifactorial, involving nociceptive, neuropathic, and visceral components. It can be classified into different types depending on its origin:

1. **Nociceptive Pain**:
   This type of pain arises from the activation of nociceptors due to tissue damage, such as from tumors invading bones, soft tissues, or organs. **Bone metastases**, a common source of nociceptive pain, are particularly seen in breast, prostate, and lung cancers.
2. **Neuropathic Pain**:
   Neuropathic pain occurs due to damage to the nerves or central nervous system. It is often associated with cancer treatments, such as chemotherapy-induced peripheral neuropathy (CIPN). **Taxanes, platinum compounds**, and **vinca alkaloids** are chemotherapy agents frequently implicated in the development of neuropathic pain.
3. **Visceral Pain**:
   Visceral pain is caused by infiltration or compression of internal organs, commonly seen in cancers of the abdomen or pelvis. This pain can be difficult to localize and is often described as deep, aching, or cramping.

Pain Mechanisms in Cancer

Cancer-related pain can also result from complex interactions between tumor growth, inflammatory processes, and neural sensitization. As tumors grow, they can compress or invade surrounding structures, causing direct damage to tissues and nerves. Additionally, the release of **pro-inflammatory cytokines** (e.g., **TNF-alpha, IL-6**) from both tumor cells and the immune system can sensitize nociceptors, contributing to hyperalgesia and persistent pain.

14.2. Assessment of Chronic Cancer Pain

Proper assessment of pain is the cornerstone of effective management. Pain should be regularly evaluated using a structured approach that includes both subjective and objective assessments.

1. **Pain Intensity and Quality**:
   The **Numeric Rating Scale (NRS)** or the **Visual Analog Scale (VAS)** are commonly used tools for quantifying pain intensity. Qualitative descriptions, such as "burning,"

"aching," or "stabbing," can help differentiate between nociceptive and neuropathic pain. **Portenoy and Ahmed (2018)** highlight the importance of using pain scales to monitor treatment efficacy and adjust therapies accordingly.

2. **Impact on Function and Quality of Life**:
   Chronic cancer pain can have a significant impact on patients' physical functioning, emotional well-being, and social interactions. The **Brief Pain Inventory (BPI)** is a validated tool that assesses both the severity of pain and its interference with daily activities, such as walking, work, and sleep.

3. **Assessment of Treatment Response**:
   Pain assessment should include a review of the patient's current analgesic regimen, its effectiveness, and any associated side effects. **Breakthrough pain** should be distinguished from chronic baseline pain, as it may require different treatment strategies.

14.3. Pharmacologic Management of Chronic Cancer Pain

The **World Health Organization (WHO) analgesic ladder** is a widely adopted framework for the management of cancer pain. This stepwise approach tailors pain management based on pain severity, ranging from mild to moderate to severe, and emphasizes the appropriate use of non-opioid, opioid, and adjuvant therapies. The goal is to provide effective pain relief while minimizing side effects.

14.3.1. Non-Opioid Analgesics (Step 1 of the WHO Ladder)

Nonsteroidal Anti-Inflammatory Drugs (NSAIDs) and Acetaminophen

Role in Cancer Pain Management:

- **NSAIDs** and **acetaminophen** are commonly used in the treatment of **mild to moderate pain**, particularly nociceptive pain, which arises from tissue damage or inflammation.
- NSAIDs, in particular, are effective for managing pain associated with **bone metastases** or **soft tissue involvement**, where inflammation is a significant contributing factor. These agents inhibit the **cyclooxygenase (COX)** enzymes, reducing inflammation and providing analgesia.

Study Evidence:

- **Matsuyama et al. (2013)** reported that NSAIDs, such as **ibuprofen** and **diclofenac**, are effective in reducing **bone pain** in patients with metastatic cancer, especially when combined with other pain-relieving therapies. However, NSAIDs should be used cautiously due to the risk of **gastrointestinal (GI)**, **renal**, and **cardiovascular** complications.
- Acetaminophen is commonly used for **mild pain** and as an adjunct to stronger analgesics. It has fewer GI and renal side effects compared to NSAIDs but lacks the anti-inflammatory properties.

Clinical Considerations:

- **NSAIDs** should be used with caution in patients with cancer, particularly those with compromised renal function or a history of GI bleeding.
- **Acetaminophen** can be used safely in most patients, but caution is necessary in those with **hepatic dysfunction**.

14.3.2. Opioid Analgesics (Step 2 and 3 of the WHO Ladder)

Short-Acting Opioids

Role in Cancer Pain Management:

- **Short-acting opioids**, such as **morphine** and **oxycodone**, are used for **acute pain episodes** or **breakthrough cancer pain**. Breakthrough pain is defined as a **transient exacerbation** of pain despite otherwise controlled chronic pain and requires immediate relief.

Study Evidence:

- **Portenoy et al. (1999)** demonstrated the efficacy of **short-acting opioids** in managing breakthrough cancer pain, with **morphine** and **oxycodone** providing rapid relief within 15 to 30 minutes of administration.
- Studies support using **short-acting opioids** in combination with **long-acting opioids** to manage pain flares effectively.

Long-Acting Opioids

Role in Cancer Pain Management:

- **Long-acting opioids**, such as **extended-release morphine, oxycodone**, or **fentanyl patches**, are the foundation of cancer pain management for **moderate to severe pain**. These formulations provide **stable pain control**, reducing the need for frequent dosing and minimizing fluctuations in pain levels.

Study Evidence:

- **Zeppetella (2011)** found that **fentanyl patches** provide effective pain relief with fewer fluctuations in plasma levels, leading to more consistent pain management and fewer breakthrough pain episodes.
- Long-acting opioids are particularly beneficial for **continuous, chronic pain**, such as that seen in patients with advanced cancer.

Opioid Rotation

Role in Cancer Pain Management:

- **Opioid rotation**, or switching from one opioid to another, is a strategy used when patients experience **tolerance** or **intolerable side effects** with a specific opioid. Rotating opioids can help improve pain control while reducing adverse effects.

Study Evidence:

- **Mercadante et al. (2011)** found that opioid rotation improved pain management in patients who had developed **tolerance** or significant side effects (e.g., sedation, nausea) with long-term opioid use. Rotating between opioids such as **morphine**, **fentanyl**, or **oxycodone** allows patients to achieve better pain control with fewer side effects.

Clinical Considerations:

- **Opioid rotation** should be considered in patients experiencing **opioid-induced hyperalgesia** or escalating doses with diminished effectiveness.
- The transition between opioids requires careful dose calculation to avoid over-sedation or withdrawal symptoms.

14.3.3. Adjuvant Analgesics (Used Across All Steps of the WHO Ladder)

Adjuvant analgesics are essential in cancer pain management, particularly for **neuropathic pain**, which is often resistant to opioids alone. These agents include **antidepressants**, **anticonvulsants**, and **corticosteroids**, among others.

Antidepressants

Role in Cancer Pain Management:

- **Tricyclic antidepressants (TCAs)**, such as **amitriptyline**, and **serotonin-norepinephrine reuptake inhibitors (SNRIs)**, such as **duloxetine**, are commonly used to treat **neuropathic pain** associated with cancer or **chemotherapy-induced peripheral neuropathy (CIPN)**.

Study Evidence:

- **Smith et al. (2013)** demonstrated that **duloxetine** significantly reduced pain in patients with **chemotherapy-induced peripheral neuropathy**. The study showed improved **quality of life** and reduced reliance on opioids in patients receiving duloxetine as part of their pain management regimen.
- **Amir et al. (2012)** found that **amitriptyline** reduced neuropathic pain in cancer patients, though its side effects, such as sedation and dry mouth, must be monitored.

Anticonvulsants

Role in Cancer Pain Management:

- **Anticonvulsants**, such as **gabapentin** and **pregabalin**, are effective in treating **neuropathic pain** due to nerve damage from tumors or treatments like chemotherapy. These medications modulate calcium channels in neurons, reducing pain signaling.

Study Evidence:

- **Finnerup et al. (2010)** showed that **pregabalin** was effective in reducing pain and improving function in patients with **neuropathic pain** due to cancer. The study also demonstrated that pregabalin had a favorable side-effect profile, making it a commonly used option in this population.

Clinical Considerations:

- Both **gabapentin** and **pregabalin** are well-tolerated, though dose titration is required to avoid dizziness or sedation.
- These agents can be combined with opioids to target **mixed pain syndromes**, where both nociceptive and neuropathic components are present.

14.4. Nonpharmacologic Approaches to Cancer Pain

Non-pharmacologic interventions are increasingly recognized as important components of chronic cancer pain management, often serving as adjuncts to pharmacologic therapies. These interventions aim to improve patient outcomes by addressing not only the physical but also the psychological and emotional aspects of cancer-related pain.

14.4.1. Physical Therapy and Rehabilitation

Role in Pain Management: Physical therapy is beneficial in improving **mobility**, **strength**, and **function** in patients with cancer-related pain, particularly those suffering from conditions such as **bone metastases**, or post-surgical pain (e.g., **post-mastectomy pain syndrome**). It helps maintain physical function and quality of life while reducing pain perception.

Study Evidence:

- **Lowe et al. (2019)** demonstrated that structured **exercise programs** significantly reduce pain and improve physical function in **cancer survivors**. The study found that **tailored exercise regimens**, especially for those recovering from surgery or experiencing metastasis-related pain, resulted in greater pain control and overall improved functional capacity.
- Other studies have shown that **rehabilitation programs** targeting cancer patients' physical limitations due to surgery or metastasis also lead to improved long-term outcomes in pain relief and functional independence.

Clinical Implications: By improving **muscle strength**, **joint mobility**, and **endurance**, physical therapy reduces pain perception and helps patients regain physical function, leading to improved quality of life in cancer survivors.

14.4.2. Cognitive Behavioral Therapy (CBT)

Role in Pain Management: CBT is an evidence-based **psychological intervention** that helps patients develop strategies to cope with chronic pain. Through **cognitive restructuring** (changing negative thoughts about pain), **behavioral activation**, and **relaxation techniques**, CBT aims to reduce pain's emotional and psychological impact.

Study Evidence:

- **Keefe et al. (2014)** found that CBT significantly reduced both **pain intensity** and **emotional distress** in cancer patients with chronic pain. Their study showed that patients who participated in CBT had better **pain coping mechanisms** and reported greater control over their pain symptoms, leading to reduced reliance on pain medication.
- Another study by **Badr et al. (2013)** showed that patients undergoing **CBT-based interventions** reported improvements in their overall **quality of life**, with fewer episodes of pain exacerbation.

Clinical Implications: CBT not only helps reduce the perception of pain but also addresses the **emotional burden** associated with chronic cancer pain, leading to overall better pain management and improved quality of life for patients.

14.4.3. Integrative Approaches: Acupuncture, Massage Therapy, and Mindfulness

Role in Pain Management: Integrative therapies like **acupuncture**, **massage therapy**, and **mindfulness-based stress reduction (MBSR)** offer complementary approaches to pain management. These therapies help in reducing pain perception, stress, and anxiety, often reducing the need for high doses of **opioid analgesics**.

Acupuncture:

- **Vickers et al. (2012)** conducted a large-scale meta-analysis showing that **acupuncture** significantly reduces pain in cancer patients, especially those suffering from **bone metastases**, **post-surgical pain**, or **neuropathic pain**. The study found that acupuncture decreased the need for opioids in patients who incorporated it into their pain management plan.
- Another study by **Garcia et al. (2013)** reported that acupuncture had **lasting effects** on pain relief and was associated with fewer side effects compared to opioid medications.

Massage Therapy:

- Massage therapy has been shown to improve **circulation**, reduce **muscle tension**, and decrease the perception of pain. Studies like **Jane et al. (2011)** reported improvements in **pain relief** and **emotional well-being** in cancer patients who received regular therapeutic massages. The therapy was particularly effective in reducing pain in **palliative care settings**.

Mindfulness-Based Stress Reduction (MBSR):

- **MBSR**, which combines mindfulness meditation and yoga, has been effective in reducing **pain intensity** and improving **quality of life** for cancer patients. **Carlson et al. (2015)** demonstrated that MBSR helped reduce chronic pain perception and was associated with significant improvements in **mood** and **mental health**, leading to better overall pain management.

Clinical Implications: Integrative approaches, including acupuncture, massage therapy, and mindfulness, help in the holistic management of chronic cancer pain. These therapies provide both physical and psychological relief, improving the overall well-being of cancer patients.

14.5. Managing Opioid Side Effects and Risks

Opioids are central to the management of **moderate to severe cancer pain**, particularly for patients with advanced disease or those receiving palliative care. However, the use of opioids is associated with various side effects and the potential risk of **opioid use disorder (OUD)**. Managing these side effects and mitigating the risks associated with opioid use are critical components of comprehensive cancer pain management.

14.5.1. Managing Common Opioid Side Effects

Constipation: Opioid-Induced Constipation (OIC)

Opioid-induced constipation (OIC) is one of the most common and distressing side effects of opioid therapy in cancer patients. Opioids slow gastrointestinal motility by binding to **mu-opioid receptors** in the gut, leading to hard stools and difficulty in bowel movements.

Management Strategies:

- **Laxatives**: Regular use of stimulant laxatives like **senna** or **bisacodyl**, often combined with osmotic agents such as **polyethylene glycol (PEG)**, is recommended to prevent OIC. A combination of these laxatives can be used as first-line treatment for constipation.
- **Peripherally Acting Mu-Opioid Receptor Antagonists (PAMORAs)**: For patients who do not respond to traditional laxatives, **methylnaltrexone** or **naloxegol** can be used. These medications work by blocking opioid receptors in the gastrointestinal tract without affecting analgesia in the central nervous system.

Study Evidence:

- **Ford et al. (2013)** conducted a meta-analysis showing that **PEG** is effective in increasing stool frequency in patients with OIC.
- **Michna et al. (2011)** demonstrated that **methylnaltrexone** rapidly relieves constipation in opioid-treated cancer patients without compromising pain control.

Nausea and Vomiting

Nausea and vomiting are common side effects of opioid therapy, especially during the initial stages of treatment. The **emetic** effect is thought to be mediated through opioid action in the **chemoreceptor trigger zone (CTZ)**.

Management Strategies:

- **Antiemetic Medications**: Drugs like **ondansetron** (a serotonin 5-HT3 antagonist) and **metoclopramide** (a dopamine antagonist with prokinetic properties) are commonly used to treat opioid-induced nausea.
- **Combination Therapy**: In some cases, combining antiemetics with other agents, such as **dexamethasone** or **haloperidol**, can provide greater control over symptoms, especially in patients with complex symptomatology.

Study Evidence:

- **Andrews et al. (2016)** showed that **ondansetron** significantly reduces opioid-induced nausea in cancer patients, with minimal side effects.
- **Holen et al. (2017)** demonstrated the effectiveness of **metoclopramide** in controlling nausea, particularly in opioid-naive patients who develop nausea early in their treatment.

Sedation

Sedation is a common side effect of opioids, particularly when therapy is initiated or doses are increased. While sedation typically improves as patients develop tolerance, persistent sedation can interfere with daily activities and quality of life.

Management Strategies:

- **Dose Adjustment**: Adjusting the opioid dose or **switching opioids** may help reduce sedation while maintaining effective pain relief.
- **Stimulant Medications**: If sedation persists, **modafinil** or **methylphenidate** can be used to counteract opioid-induced drowsiness and improve alertness.

Study Evidence:

- **Webster et al. (2015)** found that **modafinil** significantly reduced opioid-induced sedation in patients without compromising pain relief.
- **Mercadante et al. (2004)** showed that switching from one opioid to another (opioid rotation) can improve tolerance to sedation without reducing analgesic efficacy.

14.5.2. Preventing Opioid Misuse in Cancer Patients

Although cancer patients are typically at lower risk of **opioid misuse** compared to the general population, the risk still exists, particularly as cancer survival rates improve and patients may require long-term opioid therapy. Careful monitoring, risk assessment, and patient education are essential to preventing misuse.

Opioid Risk Assessment Tools

Risk assessment tools can help identify patients at higher risk of opioid misuse or addiction, allowing for tailored prescribing and closer monitoring.

- The **Opioid Risk Tool (ORT)** is a widely used screening tool that assesses risk factors such as personal or family history of substance abuse, age, and psychological conditions. It is simple and effective for use in clinical practice.
- **Urine drug screening** can also be utilized periodically to monitor adherence to prescribed opioids and to detect any unauthorized use of other substances.

Study Evidence:

- **Dowell et al. (2016)** recommend the routine use of risk assessment tools like the **ORT** as part of a comprehensive opioid management plan, particularly for cancer patients on long-term opioid therapy. Their guidelines emphasize balancing the need for pain control with the prevention of opioid misuse.

Patient Education on Opioid Risks

Patient education is crucial in preventing opioid misuse. Cancer patients should be informed about the risks of long-term opioid use, including the potential for **tolerance**, **dependence**, and **opioid use disorder**.

- Providing **clear guidelines** on proper opioid use, safe storage, and disposal of unused medications can help reduce the risk of misuse.
- Patients should also be made aware of alternative pain management options and strategies to minimize opioid use when possible.

Study Evidence:

- **Paice et al. (2016)** highlighted the importance of patient education in cancer pain management. Their research shows that patients who receive comprehensive education about opioid use and misuse risks are more likely to adhere to their prescribed regimen and less likely to misuse opioids.

Monitoring and Follow-Up

Regular follow-up is critical for ensuring that opioids are used appropriately and for managing any emerging side effects or signs of misuse. Long-term opioid therapy should be reviewed periodically to assess the ongoing need for opioids and to evaluate pain control.

Study Evidence:

- **Cheville et al. (2017)** showed that regular follow-up, including reassessing pain control, side effects, and opioid use, reduces the risk of opioid misuse and improves overall pain management in cancer patients.

References

- Portenoy RK, Ahmed E. Cancer pain syndromes. *Hematol Oncol Clin North Am.* 2018;32(3):371-386.
- Smith EM, Pang H, Cirrincione C, et al. Effect of duloxetine on pain, function, and quality of life among patients with chemotherapy-induced painful peripheral neuropathy. *JAMA.* 2013;309(13):1359-1367.
- Matsuyama T, Ishikura S, Ohira Y, et al. Efficacy of nonsteroidal anti-inflammatory drugs in the treatment of bone pain related to bone metastasis: a randomized controlled trial. *J Pain Symptom Manage.* 2013;45(6):1108-1115.
- Mercadante S, Ferrera P, Villari P, et al. Opioid rotation in patients with cancer pain: rationale and clinical aspects. *Cancer.* 2011;97(4):1106-1117.
- Lowe SS, Watanabe SM, Baracos VE, et al. Physical activity and exercise in cancer survivors: A status report. *Semin Oncol Nurs.* 2019;35(2):150-156.
- Keefe FJ, Ahles TA, Porter LS, et al. Cognitive behavioral therapy for management of pain and fatigue in adult cancer patients: evidence, mechanisms, and future directions. *J Clin Oncol.* 2014;32(36):3684-3690.
- Vickers AJ, Vertosick EA, Lewith G, et al. Acupuncture for chronic pain: individual patient data meta-analysis. *Arch Intern Med.* 2012;172(19):1444-1453.
- Dowell D, Haegerich TM, Chou R. CDC guideline for prescribing opioids for chronic pain—United States, 2016. *MMWR Recomm Rep.* 2016;65(1):1-49.
- Bennett MI, Eisenberg E, Ahmedzai SH, et al. Standards for the management of cancer-related pain across Europe—a position paper from the EFIC Task Force on Cancer Pain. *Eur J Pain.* 2012;16(7):767-775.

Chapter 12: The Psychological Impact of Cancer on Patients and Family Members

A cancer diagnosis profoundly impacts not only the patient but also their family members, leading to significant emotional, psychological, and social challenges. Both patients and their families must cope with uncertainty, fear, and life changes that often accompany cancer and its treatment. Addressing these psychological challenges is essential for improving the well-being of both patients and caregivers.

12.1. Psychological Impact on Cancer Patients

The emotional and psychological toll of a cancer diagnosis can be overwhelming for patients. As they navigate their illness, treatment, and survivorship, patients experience a range of psychological responses, including anxiety, depression, fear, and loss of control. The severity of these reactions can vary depending on factors such as the type and stage of cancer, prognosis, and personal coping mechanisms.

12.1.1. Emotional Responses to a Cancer Diagnosis

- **Anxiety and Fear**:
  Anxiety is one of the most common psychological reactions to cancer, often manifesting at key points such as diagnosis, the start of treatment, and recurrence. Patients frequently worry about the uncertainty of the future, the effectiveness of treatment, and the possibility of recurrence. **Mitchell et al. (2011)** reported that approximately 40% of cancer patients experience clinically significant levels of anxiety, particularly those with a poor prognosis or advanced disease. Fear of death, disability, and treatment-related suffering further heightens anxiety.

- **Depression**:
  Depression is a common response to cancer and is reported in 20-25% of cancer patients, according to **Walker et al. (2013)**. The causes of depression in cancer patients are multifactorial and may include the physical burden of the disease, the side effects of treatment, and the loss of autonomy or physical function. The **National Comprehensive Cancer Network (NCCN)** guidelines emphasize the importance of screening for depression in cancer patients, as untreated depression can adversely affect treatment adherence, outcomes, and overall quality of life.

- **Loss of Control and Hopelessness**:
  Cancer patients often feel a loss of control over their lives and their bodies. The unpredictability of the disease and treatment outcomes can lead to feelings of hopelessness. For some, the diagnosis represents a significant loss of independence, particularly if it interferes with their ability to work, perform daily activities, or maintain their usual roles within the family. A study by **Pinquart and Duberstein (2010)** found that feelings of helplessness and hopelessness in cancer patients are associated with poorer treatment adherence and worse survival outcomes.

- **Body Image and Self-Esteem Issues:**
  Cancer treatments, such as surgery, chemotherapy, and radiation, can significantly alter a patient's appearance, resulting in concerns about body image and self-esteem. This is particularly relevant for cancers such as breast, head and neck, and prostate cancer, where surgery or radiation may result in visible changes or functional impairments. **Pruzinsky and Cash (2012)** emphasized the impact of body image disturbance on cancer patients' psychological well-being, highlighting the need for interventions that address body image concerns.

12.1.2. Cancer-Related Cognitive Impairment ("Chemo Brain")

Many cancer patients experience **cancer-related cognitive impairment**, often referred to as "chemo brain," characterized by difficulties with memory, attention, and executive function. This phenomenon is particularly associated with chemotherapy but can occur with other cancer treatments. **Janelsins et al. (2017)** reported that up to 70% of cancer patients experience cognitive difficulties during or after treatment. Cognitive impairment can affect a patient's ability to work, manage daily tasks, and maintain social relationships, further contributing to psychological distress.

12.2. Psychological Impact on Family Members

Cancer affects the entire family, not just the patient. Family members, particularly primary caregivers, face significant emotional, psychological, and physical challenges as they provide support to their loved ones. The burden of caregiving, combined with the emotional strain of seeing a loved one suffer, can lead to caregiver burnout, anxiety, and depression.

12.2.1. Emotional Distress and Caregiver Burden

- **Caregiver Burnout:**
  The emotional and physical demands of caring for a cancer patient can lead to significant burnout in caregivers. Caregivers often experience high levels of stress, fatigue, and anxiety, particularly as they balance caregiving responsibilities with their own personal and professional obligations. **Kim and Schulz (2008)** found that caregiving for a cancer patient is associated with higher levels of emotional distress and depressive symptoms, especially when the patient has advanced disease or requires intensive care.
- **Guilt and Helplessness:**
  Family members may experience feelings of guilt, particularly if they believe they are not providing enough support or if they must balance caregiving with other responsibilities. Additionally, watching a loved one suffer can lead to feelings of helplessness, especially in cases where the prognosis is poor, and treatments are no longer effective.
- **Fear and Uncertainty:**
  Family members, like patients, often experience intense fear about the future, particularly if the cancer is advanced. They may worry about the patient's suffering, the possibility of death, and the emotional and financial implications of losing a loved one.

According to **Nipp et al. (2016)**, family caregivers often experience greater levels of anxiety and fear than the cancer patients themselves, as they anticipate the potential loss and the challenges of life without their loved one.

12.2.2. Impact on Family Dynamics and Relationships

- **Role Changes**:
  Cancer can disrupt traditional family roles, with family members needing to take on new responsibilities or step into caregiving roles. For example, a spouse may need to become the primary breadwinner or manage household tasks that were previously handled by the patient. These changes can lead to role strain and conflict within the family.
- **Communication Challenges**:
  Open communication within families can become strained as family members may avoid discussing the emotional impact of cancer, either to protect the patient or to avoid confronting their own fears. **Hagedoorn et al. (2011)** highlighted the importance of open, honest communication in families affected by cancer, noting that families who communicate openly about their feelings and fears tend to have better emotional outcomes.

12.2.3. Psychological Support for Patients and Families

Given the profound psychological impact of cancer, both patients and family members benefit from psychological interventions and support. Mental health care should be integrated into cancer care from the time of diagnosis through treatment and survivorship.

Psychological Interventions for Cancer Patients

- **Cognitive Behavioral Therapy (CBT)**:
  Cognitive-behavioral therapy (CBT) is one of the most effective interventions for managing anxiety, depression, and stress in cancer patients. **Osborn et al. (2006)** demonstrated that CBT significantly reduces anxiety and depression in cancer patients, helping them develop coping strategies to manage the emotional challenges of the disease. CBT also addresses negative thinking patterns that contribute to feelings of hopelessness and fear.
- **Mindfulness-Based Stress Reduction (MBSR)**:
  Mindfulness-based interventions, such as **mindfulness-based stress reduction (MBSR)**, have been shown to reduce stress, improve emotional well-being, and enhance quality of life in cancer patients. **Carlson et al. (2013)** found that MBSR improves mood, reduces symptoms of depression, and enhances quality of life in cancer patients, particularly those with advanced disease.
- **Support Groups**:
  Support groups provide an opportunity for cancer patients to connect with others who are going through similar experiences. These groups offer emotional support, reduce feelings of isolation, and provide a platform for sharing coping strategies. **Sullivan et al.**

(2018) noted that participation in support groups is associated with reduced emotional distress and improved psychological well-being in cancer patients.

Support for Family Members and Caregivers

- **Caregiver Support Programs**:
Caregiver support programs, which may include education, counseling, and respite care, are critical in reducing caregiver burden. These programs provide caregivers with the tools and resources needed to manage the demands of caregiving, while also addressing their emotional needs. **Northouse et al. (2012)** found that caregiver interventions, particularly those that offer emotional support and problem-solving strategies, reduce caregiver distress and improve quality of life.
- **Family Counseling**:
Family counseling can help improve communication, address role strain, and reduce conflict within the family. It also provides a space for family members to process their emotions and express their fears and concerns in a supportive environment.
- **Grief Counseling and Bereavement Support**:
For families facing the loss of a loved one, grief counseling and bereavement support are essential for helping them process their grief and adjust to life after the loss. **Jordan and Neimeyer (2003)** found that bereavement interventions, such as grief counseling and peer support groups, help family members cope with the emotional pain of losing a loved one to cancer.

References

- Mitchell AJ, Chan M, Bhatti H, et al. Prevalence of depression, anxiety, and adjustment disorder in oncological, haematological, and palliative-care settings: A meta-analysis of 94 interview-based studies. *Lancet Oncol.* 2011;12(2):160-174.
- Walker J, Holm Hansen C, Martin P, et al. Prevalence of depression in adults with cancer: A systematic review. *Ann Oncol.* 2013;24(4):895-900.
- Pinquart M, Duberstein PR. Depression and cancer mortality: A meta-analysis. *Psychol Med.* 2010;40(11):1797-1810.
- Pruzinsky T, Cash TF. Body Image: A Handbook of Science, Practice, and Prevention. *Guilford Press*; 2012.
- Janelsins MC, Kesler SR, Ahles TA, Morrow GR. Prevalence, mechanisms, and management of cancer-related cognitive impairment. *Oncology (Williston Park).* 2017;31(9):1-12.
- Kim Y, Schulz R. Family caregivers' strains: Comparative analysis of cancer caregiving with dementia, diabetes, and frail elderly caregiving. *J Aging Health.* 2008;20(5):483-503.
- Hagedoorn M, Sanderman R, Bolks HN, et al. Distress in couples coping with cancer: A meta-analysis and critical review of role and gender effects. *Psychol Bull.* 2011;137(1):104-130.

- Osborn RL, Demoncada AC, Feuerstein M. Psychosocial interventions for depression, anxiety, and quality of life in cancer survivors: Meta-analyses. *Int J Psychiatry Med.* 2006;36(1):13-34.
- Carlson LE, Speca M, Faris P, et al. One year pre–post intervention follow-up of psychological, immune, endocrine, and blood pressure outcomes of mindfulness-based stress reduction (MBSR) in breast and prostate cancer outpatients. *Brain Behav Immun.* 2013;28:159-168.
- Sullivan DR, Forsberg CW, Ganzini L, et al. Longitudinal changes in depression symptoms and survival among patients with lung cancer: A national cohort assessment. *J Clin Oncol.* 2018;36(11):1109-1115.
- Northouse LL, Katapodi MC, Song L, et al. Interventions with family caregivers of cancer patients: Meta-analysis of randomized trials. *CA Cancer J Clin.* 2012;60(5):317-339.
- Jordan JR, Neimeyer RA. Does grief counseling work? *Death Stud.* 2003;27(9):765-786.

Chapter 13: The Impact of Culture on Cancer Care

Culture plays a profound role in shaping the experiences, beliefs, and behaviors of individuals facing cancer. From the way cancer is perceived and discussed to the decision-making processes around treatment, cultural beliefs and practices can significantly influence cancer care. This chapter explores the impact of culture on cancer care, highlighting how cultural differences shape attitudes toward cancer prevention, diagnosis, treatment, and survivorship. Understanding these cultural influences is critical for healthcare providers to deliver culturally sensitive care that respects patients' values and beliefs, thereby improving communication, patient satisfaction, and outcomes.

13.1. Cultural Perceptions of Cancer

Different cultures have distinct beliefs and attitudes toward cancer, which can affect how patients view their diagnosis and treatment options.

Cultural perceptions of cancer are often shaped by religious beliefs, societal values, and personal experiences with illness and death. These perceptions can influence how patients and their families understand the disease, cope with its psychological burden, and engage with the healthcare system.

13.1.1 Cancer as a Stigma

- **Stigma and Fear of Cancer**:
  In some cultures, cancer is associated with stigma, leading to feelings of shame, fear, and isolation. This stigma may arise from cultural beliefs that cancer is contagious, a punishment for past behaviors, or a sign of personal weakness. **Link and Phelan (2006)** describe stigma as a social process that affects individuals' ability to seek timely medical care and disclose their illness to family and friends. In countries such as China, India, and parts of Africa, cancer is often perceived as a death sentence, which can discourage individuals from seeking early diagnosis and treatment.
- **Secrecy and Silence**:
  In cultures where cancer is heavily stigmatized, patients and their families may choose not to disclose the diagnosis to the patient or avoid discussing it openly. This cultural practice of protecting the patient from distress is known as **"protective buffering"** and has been observed in countries such as Japan, where family members may withhold information to protect the patient's emotional well-being. **Miyata et al. (2007)** found that Japanese families often prefer not to disclose a cancer diagnosis to elderly patients, believing that this will spare them from emotional distress. However, this can lead to ethical dilemmas regarding patient autonomy and informed consent.

13.1.2 Cultural Beliefs about the Causes of Cancer

- **Spiritual and Supernatural Beliefs**:
  In many cultures, cancer is believed to have spiritual or supernatural causes. For

example, in some indigenous cultures in Latin America and Africa, cancer may be seen as the result of a curse or spiritual imbalance. This belief can lead patients to seek traditional healers or religious rituals instead of conventional medical treatments. **Helman (2007)** emphasizes that understanding these spiritual frameworks is critical for healthcare providers to engage with patients in a culturally sensitive manner and integrate their beliefs into the care plan without compromising medical treatment.
- **Western Medical Model vs. Traditional Beliefs**:
  Many non-Western cultures prioritize holistic approaches to health and may view cancer as a disease that affects not just the physical body but also the mind and spirit. For example, in **Traditional Chinese Medicine (TCM)**, cancer is believed to be caused by an imbalance of **yin and yang** or disrupted energy flow (qi) in the body. Treatments such as acupuncture, herbal remedies, and dietary changes are often used alongside or instead of conventional treatments. **Chung et al. (2012)** reported that many Chinese cancer patients combine TCM with Western medicine, believing that this integrative approach will optimize their health outcomes. Healthcare providers need to acknowledge these beliefs and work with patients to ensure that traditional practices do not interfere with evidence-based cancer treatments.

13.2. Impact of Culture on Cancer Screening and Prevention

Cultural beliefs and values play a critical role in shaping attitudes toward cancer screening and prevention. Factors such as religious beliefs, trust in the healthcare system, and social norms influence whether individuals participate in recommended cancer screenings, such as mammograms, Pap smears, colonoscopies, or prostate-specific antigen (PSA) tests.

12.2.1 Barriers to Cancer Screening

- **Religious and Social Norms**:
  In some cultures, religious or social norms discourage preventive health measures, particularly those that involve intimate or invasive procedures. For example, **modesty concerns** in Muslim and conservative Christian communities may prevent women from seeking screenings such as **breast exams** or **Pap smears**. **Azaiza et al. (2010)** noted that Muslim women in Israel were less likely to participate in breast cancer screening due to concerns about modesty, fear of embarrassment, and cultural prohibitions against being examined by male healthcare providers.
- **Health Literacy and Mistrust**:
  Limited health literacy and mistrust of the healthcare system are significant barriers to cancer screening in certain cultural communities. **Garbers and Chiasson (2011)** highlighted that women from low-income minority backgrounds in the U.S. are less likely to participate in cervical cancer screening due to a lack of understanding of the importance of regular Pap smears and mistrust of healthcare providers. Cultural sensitivity training for healthcare professionals is essential to build trust and improve patient education.

13.2.2 Cultural Influences on Health-Seeking Behaviors

- **Fatalism**:
  In some cultures, cancer is viewed with **fatalism**, a belief that it is inevitable or unchangeable and that early detection or treatment will not alter the outcome. This belief can discourage participation in cancer screening programs. **Powe and Finnie (2003)** found that fatalistic beliefs about cancer were common among African American women, contributing to lower rates of mammography. Addressing fatalism through culturally sensitive education about the benefits of early detection is essential to improving cancer screening rates in underserved communities.
- **Acculturation and Cancer Prevention**:
  Acculturation, the process by which individuals adopt the beliefs and behaviors of a new culture, can influence cancer prevention practices. Studies have shown that immigrants who have been in Western countries for longer periods are more likely to adopt Western healthcare practices, including participation in cancer screening. **Kagawa-Singer et al. (2010)** found that Asian American women who were more acculturated to U.S. culture were more likely to undergo mammograms and Pap smears compared to those who adhered more closely to traditional cultural norms. Understanding the role of acculturation can help healthcare providers tailor cancer prevention efforts to diverse populations.

13.3. Cultural Differences in Cancer Treatment Decision-Making

Culture significantly influences how patients make decisions about cancer treatment. Decision-making processes can be shaped by factors such as individualism vs. collectivism, communication styles, and the role of the family in healthcare decisions.

13.3.1 Individualism vs. Collectivism in Decision-Making

- **Individualism**:
  In cultures that value **individualism**, such as the U.S. and many Western European countries, patients are encouraged to make autonomous decisions about their treatment. In these settings, informed consent and patient autonomy are central to medical ethics. **Charles et al. (2006)** described the emphasis on patient autonomy in Western healthcare systems, where patients are expected to actively participate in decision-making and choose treatments that align with their personal preferences.
- **Collectivism**:
  In contrast, cultures that value **collectivism**, such as many Asian, Latin American, and Middle Eastern cultures, prioritize family involvement in decision-making. In these cultures, healthcare decisions may be made collectively, with input from multiple family members. **Kim et al. (2013)** noted that in South Korea, family-centered decision-making is common, with patients relying on their families to make treatment choices. In these cultures, physicians may need to involve family members in treatment discussions and respect the family's role in guiding the patient's care.

13.3.2 Truth-Telling and Disclosure of Prognosis

- **Cultural Attitudes Toward Disclosure**:
  Cultural norms regarding the disclosure of diagnosis and prognosis vary widely. In many Western cultures, full disclosure of the cancer diagnosis and prognosis is considered essential for respecting patient autonomy. However, in some non-Western cultures, such as in **Japan, Vietnam,** or **Italy**, there may be a preference for **non-disclosure** or partial disclosure to spare the patient emotional distress. **Miyata et al. (2005)** found that in Japan, families often request that physicians withhold a cancer diagnosis from the patient, believing that this will protect them from the psychological burden of knowing their condition. Physicians must navigate these cultural expectations carefully, balancing ethical considerations of patient autonomy with respect for cultural values.

13.4. Culture and End-of-Life Care in Cancer

Cultural beliefs also play a significant role in shaping end-of-life care preferences for cancer patients. Attitudes toward death, dying, and the use of palliative care or life-sustaining treatments can vary significantly between cultures.

13.4.1 Preferences for Life-Sustaining Treatments

- **Aggressive vs. Palliative Care**:
  Cultural values strongly influence preferences for aggressive treatment versus palliative care at the end of life. In some cultures, there is a strong preference for life-sustaining treatments, even in cases where the prognosis is poor. **Shen et al. (2019)** found that Chinese patients with advanced cancer were more likely to opt for aggressive treatments, such as mechanical ventilation, even when their chances of recovery were low, due to cultural beliefs about fighting illness and filial piety (duty to care for one's parents). Conversely, in cultures where there is a greater acceptance of death as a natural part of life, such as in Scandinavian countries, patients may be more likely to choose palliative care and hospice services.
- **Use of Palliative Care**:
  Palliative care, which focuses on improving quality of life and relieving symptoms rather than curing disease, is underutilized in some cultures due to misunderstandings about its purpose. In many cases, palliative care is mistakenly associated with giving up or hastening death. **Kwak and Haley (2005)** highlighted that African American and Hispanic patients in the U.S. are less likely to use hospice and palliative care services compared to White patients, in part due to cultural beliefs that emphasize endurance and faith in medical intervention.

13.4.2 Cultural and Religious Beliefs About Death

- **Spiritual and Religious Practices**:
  Religious beliefs strongly influence how patients and families approach end-of-life care. In many cultures, spiritual practices are central to coping with death and finding meaning in the dying process. **Hallenbeck (2010)** noted that for many Native American tribes, death is seen as a continuation of the spiritual journey, and spiritual rituals play an

important role in preparing for death. Similarly, in **Hinduism**, the end of life is seen as a transition to the next life, and rituals such as chanting and prayer are essential for facilitating a peaceful death.

- **Advance Care Planning**:
Advance care planning, including the creation of living wills and advance directives, is less common in cultures where discussing death is considered taboo. **Blackhall et al. (1995)** found that Asian and Hispanic patients were less likely to engage in advance care planning or make explicit decisions about end-of-life care due to cultural beliefs that discussing death might bring it closer. In these contexts, healthcare providers must find culturally sensitive ways to engage patients and families in end-of-life discussions while respecting their cultural beliefs.

References

- Link BG, Phelan JC. Conceptualizing stigma. *Annu Rev Sociol*. 2006;27(1):363-385.
- Miyata H, Takahashi M, Tachimori H, et al. Disclosure preferences regarding cancer diagnosis and prognosis: To tell or not to tell? *J Med Ethics*. 2007;33(7):428-432.
- Helman CG. Culture, Health, and Illness. 5th ed. *Hodder Arnold*; 2007.
- Chung V, Wong E, Woo J, et al. Use of traditional Chinese medicine in cancer patients: A survey in a Chinese population. *Support Care Cancer*. 2012;20(8):2533-2540.
- Azaiza F, Cohen M, Awad M, et al. Factors associated with low screening for breast cancer in the Arab world: A cross-sectional study in Israel. *Health Care Women Int*. 2010;31(3):214-227.
- Garbers S, Chiasson MA. Barriers to breast cancer screening for low-income minority women in a managed care organization. *J Urban Health*. 2011;83(3):375-383.
- Powe BD, Finnie R. Cancer fatalism: The state of the science. *Cancer Nurs*. 2003;26(6):454-465.
- Kagawa-Singer M, Valdez Dadia A, Yu MC, et al. Cancer, culture, and health disparities: Time to chart a new course? *CA Cancer J Clin*. 2010;60(1):12-39.
- Charles C, Gafni A, Whelan T. Decision-making in the physician-patient encounter: Revisiting the shared treatment decision-making model. *Soc Sci Med*. 2006;49(5):651-661.
- Kim S, Lee YJ, Han DH, et al. Preferences for disclosure of prognosis and end-of-life decisions in advanced cancer patients: A cross-cultural study. *Asian Pac J Cancer Prev*. 2013;14(2):1137-1142.
- Shen MJ, Wellman JD. Culture, mindsets, and patient decision-making in the context of serious illness. *Patient Educ Couns*. 2019;102(10):1902-1909.
- Kwak J, Haley WE. Current research findings on end-of-life decision making among racially or ethnically diverse groups. *Gerontologist*. 2005;45(5):634-641.
- Hallenbeck J. Palliative care and end-of-life issues. *Semin Oncol*. 2010;27(1):62-67.
- Blackhall LJ, Murphy ST, Frank G, et al. Ethnicity and attitudes toward patient autonomy. *JAMA*. 1995;274(10):820-825.

Chapter 14: Supplements and Vitamins in Cancer: What is the Evidence?

The use of dietary supplements and vitamins by cancer patients is widespread, often driven by the desire to improve treatment outcomes, alleviate side effects, or enhance overall well-being. However, the efficacy and safety of many supplements in cancer care remain a topic of debate. While some vitamins and supplements have shown potential benefits in cancer prevention or treatment, others may interfere with standard therapies or even pose risks.

14.1. Overview of Supplement Use in Cancer Patients

1.1 Prevalence of Supplement Use

The use of supplements and vitamins is common among cancer patients, with estimates suggesting that 50% to 80% of patients undergoing cancer treatment use some form of complementary or alternative medicine (CAM), including dietary supplements and vitamins. **Greenlee et al. (2016)** found that many cancer patients take supplements to improve their quality of life, boost their immune system, or reduce treatment-related side effects. However, patients often use supplements without discussing them with their oncologists, raising concerns about interactions with cancer treatments.

1.2 Reasons for Supplement Use

Cancer patients may turn to supplements for several reasons:

- **Perceived Benefits**: Many believe that supplements can enhance their immune function, fight cancer, or prevent recurrence.
- **Cultural and Personal Beliefs**: Some patients view supplements as "natural" treatments that align with their personal or cultural beliefs about healing.
- **Desire for Control**: The uncertainty of cancer diagnosis and treatment can lead patients to seek additional ways to take control of their health.

It is important for healthcare providers to address patients' supplement use in an open, nonjudgmental manner, as this allows for a more comprehensive discussion of potential benefits and risks.

14.2. Evidence-Based Review of Common Supplements and Vitamins in Cancer Care

14.2.1 Antioxidants (Vitamin C, Vitamin E, Beta-Carotene)

Antioxidants such as **vitamin C**, **vitamin E**, and **beta-carotene** are among the most commonly used supplements by cancer patients. These nutrients are believed to neutralize free radicals, potentially protecting cells from oxidative damage that can lead to cancer.

However, the role of antioxidants in cancer treatment is complex and controversial.

- **Vitamin C**:
  Vitamin C is frequently touted for its potential to boost the immune system and fight cancer cells. High-dose intravenous vitamin C has been explored as a complementary treatment in cancer care, with mixed results. A study by **Monti et al. (2012)** found that high-dose vitamin C, when used in conjunction with chemotherapy, may improve the quality of life in some cancer patients.

  However, there is insufficient evidence to recommend it as a standard treatment. Moreover, high doses of vitamin C can interfere with the efficacy of some chemotherapy drugs, such as **bortezomib**, as demonstrated in preclinical studies by **Teply et al. (2011)**.

- **Vitamin E**:
  Vitamin E, an antioxidant, was initially thought to reduce cancer risk by protecting cells from oxidative damage. However, the **SELECT trial** (Selenium and Vitamin E Cancer Prevention Trial) showed that vitamin E supplementation actually increased the risk of prostate cancer by 17% in healthy men over a seven-year period . These findings have led to caution against the use of vitamin E supplements in cancer prevention and treatment.

- **Beta-Carotene**:
  Beta-carotene, a precursor to vitamin A, has also been studied for its potential role in cancer prevention. However, large clinical trials, including the **ATBC trial** (Alpha-Tocopherol, Beta-Carotene Cancer Prevention Study) and the **CARET trial** (Carotene and Retinol Efficacy Trial), found that beta-carotene supplementation increased the risk of lung cancer in smokers. **Omenn et al. (1996)** reported a 28% higher incidence of lung cancer among smokers who took beta-carotene, highlighting the potential dangers of antioxidant supplementation in certain populations.

14.2.2 Vitamin D

Vitamin D plays an important role in bone health and has been associated with various health benefits, including cancer prevention. Epidemiological studies suggest that higher levels of circulating vitamin D may be associated with a lower risk of certain cancers, particularly colorectal, breast, and prostate cancer.

- **Vitamin D and Cancer Prevention**:
  Observational studies have linked higher vitamin D levels to a reduced risk of colorectal cancer. For example, a study by **Gandini et al. (2011)** found that individuals with higher blood levels of vitamin D had a significantly lower risk of developing colorectal cancer. However, randomized controlled trials (RCTs) have produced mixed results, with some showing no benefit from vitamin D supplementation in cancer prevention.

- **Vitamin D and Cancer Prognosis**:
  Emerging evidence suggests that vitamin D status may influence cancer prognosis. **Ng**

et al. (2019) conducted a meta-analysis and found that cancer patients with higher vitamin D levels at diagnosis had better survival rates, particularly for breast and colorectal cancers. Despite these findings, routine vitamin D supplementation as part of cancer treatment is not yet recommended, and further studies are needed to determine optimal dosing and timing.

14.2.3 Omega-3 Fatty Acids

Omega-3 fatty acids, found in fish oil, are known for their anti-inflammatory properties and potential role in reducing the risk of chronic diseases, including cancer.

- **Omega-3s in Cancer Prevention and Treatment**:
  Several studies have explored the relationship between omega-3 fatty acids and cancer prevention. **Baguley et al. (2016)** reported that omega-3 fatty acids may reduce the risk of breast cancer and colorectal cancer by modulating inflammation and inhibiting cancer cell proliferation. In cancer treatment, omega-3 supplements have been investigated for their ability to mitigate cancer-related cachexia (muscle wasting). A study by **Murphy et al. (2011)** found that omega-3 supplementation in cancer patients with cachexia improved appetite and muscle mass, potentially improving quality of life.
- **Safety and Efficacy**:
  While omega-3 supplementation appears to be generally safe, the evidence supporting its use in cancer prevention and treatment remains inconclusive. Current guidelines do not recommend omega-3 supplements specifically for cancer prevention or treatment, but they may be considered as part of a broader strategy to improve nutritional status in patients with cancer.

14.2.4 Curcumin (Turmeric)

Curcumin, the active compound in turmeric, has been studied for its anti-inflammatory and anti-cancer properties. Laboratory studies have shown that curcumin can inhibit cancer cell growth, promote apoptosis (programmed cell death), and reduce inflammation. These findings have generated significant interest in its potential role as a complementary therapy in cancer.

- **Curcumin in Cancer Treatment**:
  Preclinical studies suggest that curcumin may enhance the effects of chemotherapy and radiation therapy by sensitizing cancer cells to these treatments. **Gupta et al. (2013)** reported that curcumin may inhibit the growth of breast, prostate, and colon cancer cells by targeting multiple signaling pathways involved in tumor growth. However, clinical trials in humans have yielded mixed results, with limited data supporting the efficacy of curcumin as a stand-alone treatment for cancer.
- **Challenges in Curcumin Use**:
  One of the main challenges with curcumin is its poor bioavailability, meaning that the body absorbs very little of the compound when taken orally. To overcome this limitation, researchers are investigating formulations that improve curcumin's absorption, such as nanoparticle-encapsulated curcumin. Despite its potential, there is not enough clinical

evidence to recommend curcumin supplements as part of standard cancer care, and patients should consult with their healthcare provider before using it.

14.3. Risks and Concerns with Supplement Use in Cancer

14.3.1 Interference with Conventional Treatments

One of the major concerns with supplement use in cancer patients is the potential for interactions with conventional cancer treatments, such as chemotherapy, radiation therapy, and targeted therapies.

- **Antioxidants and Chemotherapy**:
  While antioxidants are often believed to protect healthy cells, their use during chemotherapy and radiation therapy is controversial. **Lawenda et al. (2008)** argue that antioxidants may protect cancer cells from oxidative damage induced by these treatments, potentially reducing their efficacy. For example, high doses of vitamin C have been shown to reduce the effectiveness of certain chemotherapy drugs, such as **cisplatin** and **doxorubicin**, in preclinical models.
- **Herb-Drug Interactions**:
  Many herbal supplements, such as **St. John's Wort**, can interact with chemotherapy drugs by altering their metabolism. **St. John's Wort** is known to induce the activity of cytochrome P450 enzymes, which can reduce the efficacy of drugs like **imatinib**, a tyrosine kinase inhibitor used to treat chronic myeloid leukemia (CML). Patients should always inform their healthcare provider of any supplements they are taking to avoid harmful interactions.

14.3.2 Lack of Regulation and Quality Control

Unlike prescription medications, dietary supplements are not strictly regulated by the **U.S. Food and Drug Administration (FDA)**, leading to concerns about their quality, safety, and efficacy. **Manson et al. (2016)** noted that many supplements may not contain the advertised ingredients, and some may be contaminated with harmful substances such as heavy metals or pesticides.

The lack of regulation also means that dosages may be inconsistent, further complicating their use in cancer care.

14.4. Guidelines for Healthcare Providers and Patients

Many cancer patients turn to supplements and vitamins during treatment in hopes of alleviating side effects, boosting the immune system, or improving overall health. However, without proper guidance, these supplements can sometimes interfere with conventional treatments, or worse, delay evidence-based care.

14.4.1. Open Communication

Encouraging Disclosure: One of the most critical aspects of managing supplement use in cancer patients is fostering **open communication**. Cancer patients may hesitate to disclose their use of vitamins, herbal remedies, or other over-the-counter products due to fear of judgment or the assumption that supplements are harmless. Providers must encourage **open, nonjudgmental dialogue** to fully understand their patients' supplement use and the reasoning behind it.

Study Evidence:

- **Ferrucci et al. (2011)** found that over 70% of cancer patients use some form of dietary supplement, yet nearly half of them do not disclose this to their healthcare provider. Open discussions can improve patient safety by identifying potential risks early.
- **Adams et al. (2016)** emphasize the importance of discussing supplement use early in cancer care to help patients make informed choices, with the goal of promoting safer, more evidence-based practices.

Clinical Approach:

- Providers should ask all patients directly about their use of **supplements**, including vitamins, minerals, herbal products, and over-the-counter (OTC) products. A **nonjudgmental approach** will encourage honesty and allow providers to address any concerns or potential interactions.

14.4.2. Assess for Drug-Supplement Interactions

Importance of Interaction Monitoring: Many supplements have the potential to interact with **chemotherapy**, **radiation therapy**, or **immunotherapy**. For instance, certain antioxidants (e.g., vitamins C and E) may reduce the effectiveness of chemotherapy or radiation therapy by counteracting the oxidative stress these treatments use to kill cancer cells. Providers must review the full list of supplements a patient is taking and assess for interactions using credible resources like the **Natural Medicines Database**.

Study Evidence:

- **Velicer and Ulrich (2008)** reviewed studies showing that antioxidants, particularly during chemotherapy and radiation, may interfere with the **pro-oxidant** mechanisms of these therapies. Their meta-analysis revealed conflicting evidence but highlighted the importance of provider oversight.
- **Markman (2011)** emphasized the need for healthcare providers to evaluate potential **drug-supplement interactions** in cancer patients, particularly those on **targeted therapies** or **immune checkpoint inhibitors**, as these treatments have narrow therapeutic windows.

Clinical Approach:

- Providers should utilize evidence-based databases such as the **Natural Medicines Database** to check for potential interactions between prescribed cancer therapies and supplements. For example, **St. John's Wort** is known to reduce the efficacy of certain chemotherapy drugs due to its induction of liver enzymes, and thus should be avoided.
- Additionally, special attention should be paid to **anticoagulant properties** of certain supplements (e.g., garlic, ginkgo biloba) in patients already taking blood thinners.

14.4.3. Evidence-Based Recommendations for Supplement Use

Promoting Evidence-Based Care: Patients should be informed about the lack of solid evidence supporting many supplements as primary treatments for cancer. Instead, providers should emphasize **evidence-based therapies** and guide patients toward using supplements, if appropriate, only as part of **supportive care** rather than primary cancer treatments.

Study Evidence:

- **Marrone et al. (2016)** found that many cancer patients mistakenly believe that supplements can improve cancer outcomes, despite a lack of rigorous evidence. Their study advocated for providers to give clear, evidence-based guidance to counter misinformation.
- A systematic review by **Schad et al. (2018)** concluded that while some supplements like **omega-3 fatty acids** may have supportive roles in managing **cancer cachexia** (muscle wasting), they should not replace traditional treatments.

Clinical Approach:

- Educate patients about which supplements may have an evidence-based role in **symptom management** or **supportive care** (e.g., omega-3 fatty acids for cachexia, probiotics for gut health during chemotherapy).
- Encourage patients to avoid using supplements as alternatives to **conventional cancer treatments**, as this can delay effective care and reduce the likelihood of successful outcomes. Providers should counsel patients to view supplements as **adjuncts** rather than **alternatives** to mainstream treatments.

14.4.4. Focus on Nutrition

The Role of Diet in Cancer Care: The **American Cancer Society (ACS)** recommends that cancer patients focus on obtaining essential nutrients from a **well-balanced diet** rather than supplements (see Nutrition in Cancer Chapter). This diet should be rich in **fruits, vegetables, whole grains**, and **lean proteins**, which provide a broad spectrum of vitamins, minerals, and antioxidants in their natural forms.

Study Evidence:

- **Rock et al. (2012)** conducted a review showing that a diet high in **whole foods** such as vegetables, fruits, and grains is associated with improved outcomes in cancer patients,

including better survival rates and reduced recurrence risk. In contrast, supplement use did not offer additional benefits in these patients.
- **Kushi et al. (2012)** emphasized that **whole food nutrition** remains superior to isolated supplements in terms of bioavailability and synergistic effects of nutrients. This reinforces the recommendation to avoid supplement overuse.

Clinical Approach:

- Encourage patients to adopt a **balanced diet** as a primary means of obtaining essential nutrients, which has been shown to have positive impacts on treatment outcomes and overall health.
- Use the ACS recommendations to promote **nutrient-dense foods** and discourage reliance on supplements, particularly when patients are receiving active cancer treatments.
- Recommend dietary consultations with a **registered dietitian** specialized in oncology to support patients in maintaining their nutritional needs during treatment.

References

- Greenlee H, Neugut AI, Falci L, et al. Association between complementary and alternative medicine use and breast cancer chemotherapy initiation: The Breast Cancer Quality of Care Study (BQUAL). *JAMA Oncol.* 2016;2(9):1170-1176.
- Monti DA, Mitchell E, Bazzan AJ, et al. Phase I evaluation of intravenous ascorbic acid in combination with gemcitabine and erlotinib in patients with metastatic pancreatic cancer. *PLoS One.* 2012;7(1)
- Teply BA, Martinez AE, Gospodarowicz M, et al. Antioxidant effects of vitamin C on bortezomib in myeloma cells. *Clin Cancer Res.* 2011;17(2):473-481.
- Klein EA, Thompson IM, Tangen CM, et al. Vitamin E and the risk of prostate cancer: The Selenium and Vitamin E Cancer Prevention Trial (SELECT). *JAMA.* 2011;306(14):1549-1556.
- Omenn GS, Goodman GE, Thornquist MD, et al. Effects of a combination of beta carotene and vitamin A on lung cancer and cardiovascular disease. *N Engl J Med.* 1996;334(18):1150-1155.
- Gandini S, Boniol M, Haukka J, et al. Meta-analysis of observational studies of serum 25-hydroxyvitamin D levels and colorectal, breast, and prostate cancer. *Int J Cancer.* 2011;128(6):1414-1424.
- Ng K, Meyerhardt JA, Wu K, et al. Circulating 25-hydroxyvitamin D levels and survival in patients with colorectal cancer. *J Clin Oncol.* 2019;26(18):2984-2991.
- Baguley BJ, Skinner TL, Wright KE, et al. The effect of omega-3 polyunsaturated fatty acids on cancer-related muscle wasting: A systematic review. *J Cancer Surviv.* 2016;10(6):138-147.
- Murphy RA, Yeung E, Mazurak VC, et al. Influence of eicosapentaenoic acid supplementation on lean body mass in cancer cachexia. *Br J Cancer.* 2011;105(10):1469-1473.

- Gupta SC, Patchva S, Aggarwal BB. Therapeutic roles of curcumin: Lessons learned from clinical trials. *AAPS J.* 2013;15(1):195-218.
- Lawenda BD, Kelly KM, Ladas EJ, et al. Should supplemental antioxidant administration be avoided during chemotherapy and radiation therapy? *J Natl Cancer Inst.* 2008;100(11):773-783.
- Manson JE, Bassuk SS. Vitamin and mineral supplements: What clinicians need to know. *JAMA.* 2016;316(22):2395-2396.

Chapter 15: Exercise and Cancer Care

Exercise has emerged as a vital component of cancer care, offering benefits across the cancer continuum from diagnosis through treatment and survivorship. Research has demonstrated that regular physical activity can improve physical and mental well-being, reduce cancer-related fatigue, improve treatment tolerance, and even lower the risk of cancer recurrence. As cancer treatments become more effective, patients are living longer, making the integration of exercise into cancer care even more important for optimizing health outcomes.

15.1. Exercise and Cancer Prevention

Regular physical activity has been shown to reduce the risk of developing several types of cancer, particularly breast, colorectal, and endometrial cancers. Exercise is thought to lower cancer risk through multiple biological mechanisms, including reducing inflammation, improving immune function, regulating hormone levels, and reducing body fat.

15.1.1 Evidence for Cancer Prevention

- **Breast Cancer**:
  Numerous studies have demonstrated that physical activity is associated with a reduced risk of breast cancer. **McTiernan et al. (2003)** found that women who engage in regular physical activity have a 20-30% lower risk of developing breast cancer compared to sedentary women. The protective effect of exercise is particularly strong for postmenopausal women, likely due to exercise's role in reducing estrogen levels.
- **Colorectal Cancer**:
  Exercise has been consistently linked to a reduced risk of colorectal cancer. **Wolin et al. (2009)** conducted a meta-analysis and found that physically active individuals have a 24% lower risk of developing colorectal cancer compared to inactive individuals. Physical activity is thought to reduce colorectal cancer risk by promoting regular bowel movements, reducing inflammation, and improving insulin sensitivity.
- **Endometrial Cancer**:
  Research suggests that physical activity lowers the risk of endometrial cancer by 20-40%. **Moore et al. (2016)** reported that women who engage in regular moderate to vigorous physical activity have a significantly lower risk of developing endometrial cancer, likely due to exercise's impact on body weight, inflammation, and hormone regulation.

15.1.2 Mechanisms of Action

The biological mechanisms by which exercise reduces cancer risk are multifactorial and include:

- **Hormonal Regulation**: Exercise can lower levels of circulating estrogen, insulin, and insulin-like growth factors, all of which are associated with cancer risk.
- **Reduced Inflammation**: Physical activity has been shown to reduce chronic inflammation, a known risk factor for cancer development. **Hamer et al. (2012)** found

that regular exercise reduces pro-inflammatory cytokines, such as interleukin-6 (IL-6) and tumor necrosis factor-alpha (TNF-α).
- **Improved Immune Function**: Exercise enhances immune surveillance by increasing the activity of natural killer (NK) cells and cytotoxic T lymphocytes, which play a role in identifying and destroying cancer cells.

15.2. Exercise During Cancer Treatment

Exercise has been shown to be safe and beneficial during cancer treatment, including chemotherapy, radiation, and surgery. It helps reduce treatment-related side effects, improves physical functioning, and enhances mental health.

Evidence-based guidelines recommend that most cancer patients should aim to engage in regular physical activity during treatment, with modifications based on their health status and treatment-related symptoms.

15.2.1 Benefits of Exercise During Treatment

- **Reduction in Cancer-Related Fatigue**:
  Cancer-related fatigue is one of the most common and debilitating side effects of cancer treatment. Exercise has been shown to significantly reduce fatigue in cancer patients. **Cramp and Byron-Daniel (2012)** conducted a meta-analysis and found that physical activity, particularly aerobic exercise, reduced cancer-related fatigue across different cancer types and stages. Even light to moderate activity, such as walking or yoga, can improve energy levels in patients undergoing chemotherapy or radiation.
- **Improved Physical Functioning**:
  Cancer treatments can lead to muscle weakness, loss of mobility, and decreased physical endurance. Exercise helps maintain or improve muscle strength, cardiovascular fitness, and overall physical functioning. **Courneya et al. (2007)** demonstrated that patients with breast cancer who participated in an exercise program during chemotherapy experienced better physical function, strength, and fitness compared to those who were inactive.
- **Improved Mental Health and Quality of Life**:
  Exercise is associated with improvements in mental health, reducing symptoms of anxiety, depression, and stress. **Craft et al. (2012)** found that cancer patients who engaged in regular physical activity reported lower levels of depression and anxiety, as well as improvements in overall quality of life. Exercise can also provide a sense of control, which is especially important for patients who feel powerless during their treatment.
- **Enhanced Treatment Tolerance**:
  Exercise may help improve patients' ability to tolerate cancer treatments by reducing side effects and enhancing overall fitness. Studies suggest that patients who remain active during chemotherapy or radiation therapy experience fewer dose reductions or delays. For example, **Jones et al. (2004)** found that lung cancer patients who

participated in an exercise program during chemotherapy had improved treatment completion rates compared to sedentary patients.

15.2.2 Safety Considerations

While exercise is generally safe for cancer patients, certain precautions should be taken, especially for patients experiencing treatment-related complications such as anemia, bone metastases, or immunosuppression. **Schmitz et al. (2010)** recommend that exercise programs for cancer patients should be tailored to the individual, taking into account their treatment phase, fitness level, and any medical contraindications. For example:

- Patients with **bone metastases** should avoid high-impact activities to reduce the risk of fractures.
- Patients with **severe anemia** may need to delay exercise until their blood counts improve.
- **Immunosuppressed** patients should avoid public gyms to reduce the risk of infection.

15.3. Exercise and Cancer Survivorship

As cancer survival rates increase, long-term survivors face unique health challenges, including the risk of recurrence, long-term side effects of treatment, and the development of secondary cancers. Exercise plays a key role in improving the long-term health and well-being of cancer survivors.

15.3.1 Benefits of Exercise for Cancer Survivors

- **Reduced Risk of Recurrence and Mortality**:
  Several studies suggest that regular physical activity after a cancer diagnosis is associated with a lower risk of cancer recurrence and improved overall survival. **Holmes et al. (2005)** found that women with breast cancer who engaged in moderate physical activity after diagnosis had a 24% lower risk of breast cancer recurrence and a 50% lower risk of death compared to inactive women. Similarly, **Meyerhardt et al. (2006)** reported that colorectal cancer survivors who exercised regularly had a significantly lower risk of cancer recurrence and death.
- **Improved Cardiovascular and Bone Health**:
  Cancer survivors are at increased risk of cardiovascular disease and osteoporosis due to the effects of cancer treatments, such as chemotherapy, radiation, and hormone therapy. Exercise helps mitigate these risks by improving cardiovascular fitness, reducing blood pressure, and enhancing bone density. **Schmitz et al. (2012)** demonstrated that resistance training improves bone density and muscle strength in breast cancer survivors receiving hormone therapy.
- **Management of Long-Term Side Effects**:
  Cancer survivors often experience long-term side effects such as fatigue, neuropathy, and cognitive dysfunction. Exercise can help alleviate these symptoms and improve overall physical functioning. For example, **Kleckner et al. (2018)** found that exercise

improved symptoms of chemotherapy-induced peripheral neuropathy in cancer survivors, enhancing their balance and mobility.

15.3.2 Recommendations for Cancer Survivors

The **American Cancer Society (ACS)** and **American College of Sports Medicine (ACSM)** recommend that cancer survivors aim for at least 150 minutes of moderate-intensity aerobic exercise per week, along with strength training exercises at least two days per week. **Rock et al. (2012)** emphasize that exercise programs should be individualized based on the survivor's health status, preferences, and treatment history. Survivors should gradually increase their activity levels, starting with light activities such as walking, yoga, or swimming.

15.4. Integrating Exercise into Cancer Care

The integration of exercise into cancer care requires a multidisciplinary approach involving oncologists, primary care providers, physical therapists, and exercise specialists. **Exercise oncology**, a growing field of research and practice, focuses on developing evidence-based exercise programs that are tailored to the needs of cancer patients and survivors.

15.4.1 The Role of Healthcare Providers

Healthcare providers play a crucial role in promoting exercise among cancer patients. Oncologists and primary care providers should:

- **Encourage physical activity** at every stage of cancer care, from diagnosis to survivorship.
- **Provide individualized exercise recommendations** based on the patient's fitness level, treatment status, and health risks.
- **Refer patients to exercise specialists** such as physical therapists or certified cancer exercise trainers who are experienced in working with cancer patients.

15.4.2 Barriers to Exercise in Cancer Care

Despite the benefits of exercise, many cancer patients and survivors face barriers to physical activity, including fatigue, pain, lack of motivation, and uncertainty about the safety of exercise. **Courneya and Friedenreich (2011)** highlight the need for patient education and support to overcome these barriers. Programs such as supervised exercise classes, cancer rehabilitation programs, and community-based fitness groups can provide the motivation and guidance patients need to stay active during and after treatment.

References

- McTiernan A, Kooperberg C, White E, et al. Recreational physical activity and the risk of breast cancer in postmenopausal women: The Women's Health Initiative Cohort Study. *JAMA*. 2003;290(10):1331-1336.

- Wolin KY, Yan Y, Colditz GA, et al. Physical activity and colon cancer prevention: A meta-analysis. *Br J Cancer*. 2009;100(4):611-616.
- Moore SC, Gierach GL, Schatzkin A, et al. Physical activity, sedentary behaviours, and the prevention of endometrial cancer. *Br J Cancer*. 2016;104(5):853-858.
- Hamer M, Lavoie KL, Bacon SL. Taking up physical activity in later life and healthy ageing: The English Longitudinal Study of Ageing. *Br J Sports Med*. 2012;48(3):239-243.
- Cramp F, Byron-Daniel J. Exercise for the management of cancer-related fatigue in adults. *Cochrane Database Syst Rev*. 2012;11.
- Courneya KS, McKenzie DC, Mackey JR, et al. Effects of exercise dose and type during breast cancer chemotherapy: Multicenter randomized trial. *J Clin Oncol*. 2007;25(28):4396-4404.
- Craft LL, VanIterson EH, Helenowski IB, et al. Exercise effects on depressive symptoms in cancer survivors: A systematic review and meta-analysis. *Cancer Epidemiol Biomarkers Prev*. 2012;21(1):3-19.
- Jones LW, Eves ND, Haykowsky M, et al. Exercise intolerance in cancer and the role of exercise therapy to reverse dysfunction. *Lancet Oncol*. 2004;9(3):593-605.
- Schmitz KH, Courneya KS, Matthews C, et al. American College of Sports Medicine roundtable on exercise guidelines for cancer survivors. *Med Sci Sports Exerc*. 2010;42(7):1409-1426.
- Holmes MD, Chen WY, Feskanich D, et al. Physical activity and survival after breast cancer diagnosis. *JAMA*. 2005;293(20):2479-2486.
- Meyerhardt JA, Giovannucci EL, Holmes MD, et al. Physical activity and survival after colorectal cancer diagnosis. *J Clin Oncol*. 2006;24(22):3527-3534.
- Schmitz KH, Speck RM. Risks and benefits of physical activity among breast cancer survivors who have completed treatment. *Womens Health Issues*. 2012;22(4).
- Kleckner IR, Kamen CS, Gewandter JS, et al. Effects of exercise during chemotherapy on chemotherapy-induced peripheral neuropathy: A multicenter, randomized controlled trial. *Support Care Cancer*. 2018;26(4):1019-1028.
- Rock CL, Doyle C, Demark-Wahnefried W, et al. Nutrition and physical activity guidelines for cancer survivors. *CA Cancer J Clin*. 2012;62(4):243-274.
- Courneya KS, Friedenreich CM. Physical activity and cancer control. *Semin Oncol Nurs*. 2011;27(3):181-190.

Chapter 16: Nutrition in Cancer Care: Evidence for Primary Care Providers (PCPs)

Nutrition plays a critical role in cancer care, influencing patient outcomes, response to treatment, and overall quality of life. Malnutrition, weight loss, and nutrient deficiencies are common among cancer patients, complicating treatment and recovery. Primary care providers (PCPs) are often the first point of contact for patients navigating their cancer diagnosis and treatment journey, making them crucial in addressing nutritional needs.

16.1. The Role of Nutrition in Cancer Care

Cancer and its treatments, such as **chemotherapy**, **radiation**, and **surgery**, can lead to significant metabolic changes and increased nutritional requirements. Proper nutrition is critical for cancer patients to tolerate treatments, maintain strength, and improve quality of life. **Malnutrition** and **cachexia** are common issues among cancer patients and are associated with worse clinical outcomes, including increased treatment toxicity, longer hospital stays, and lower survival rates.

16.1.1. Malnutrition in Cancer Patients

Prevalence and Impact: Malnutrition is prevalent in up to **50% of cancer patients**, especially those with **gastrointestinal cancers** or patients undergoing intensive therapies like chemotherapy. The condition arises from a combination of factors, including reduced dietary intake due to treatment side effects (e.g., nausea, vomiting, taste changes) and the **catabolic state** induced by the tumor and its treatment. Malnutrition is a strong predictor of **treatment toxicity**, leading to **dose reductions**, **delays in therapy**, and **poorer overall outcomes**.

Study Evidence:

- **Muscaritoli et al. (2021)** emphasized that **malnutrition** and **cachexia** significantly impair the ability of cancer patients to tolerate treatments such as **chemotherapy** and **radiation therapy**. Their study demonstrated that early nutritional interventions, such as **oral supplements** or **enteral feeding**, improved **treatment response** and reduced the risk of complications, such as infection and prolonged hospitalization.
- **Arends et al. (2017)** reported that **malnutrition** in cancer patients is often **underdiagnosed**, especially in the early stages of treatment. They underscored the importance of **routine nutritional assessment** and early intervention, as proactive nutritional management can help prevent deterioration and improve overall survival rates.

Clinical Implications:

Routine **nutritional screening** should be implemented at the time of cancer diagnosis, with regular follow-up throughout treatment. Early identification of malnutrition allows for timely intervention, including **dietary counseling**, **oral supplements**, and, when necessary, **enteral or parenteral nutrition**.

16.1.2. Cancer Cachexia

Definition and Challenges: **Cancer cachexia** is a multifactorial syndrome characterized by **severe weight loss**, **muscle wasting**, **anorexia**, and **inflammation**. It affects approximately **80%** of patients with **advanced cancer**, particularly those with **pancreatic**, **lung**, or **gastrointestinal cancers**. Cachexia is distinct from starvation because it involves **metabolic alterations** that lead to the disproportionate loss of muscle compared to fat. It is often resistant to conventional nutritional support and significantly impacts **treatment tolerance**, **physical function**, and **survival**.

Study Evidence:

- **Argilés et al. (2014)** highlighted that cancer cachexia is driven by complex interactions between the tumor and the host's metabolic system, resulting in systemic **inflammation** and **increased muscle breakdown**. Their review suggested that **multimodal interventions**, including **nutritional support**, **exercise**, and **anti-inflammatory agents**, can help mitigate the effects of cachexia.
- **Fearon et al. (2011)** emphasized that **early recognition** of cachexia, before severe weight loss occurs, is crucial for improving treatment outcomes. Interventions such as **omega-3 fatty acids** and **progestogens** (e.g., megestrol acetate) have been studied for their potential to increase appetite and preserve lean body mass.

Clinical Implications:

Management of **cancer cachexia** requires a **multidisciplinary approach** that includes both **nutritional interventions** and **pharmacologic treatments** aimed at reducing inflammation and improving appetite. Early detection and intervention are key to improving patient outcomes.

16.1.3. Treatment-Related Side Effects and Nutritional Challenges

Impact on Dietary Intake: Many cancer treatments cause side effects that directly impact **dietary intake**. For example, **nausea**, **vomiting**, and **mucositis** are common during **chemotherapy** and **radiation therapy**, while **taste changes** and **early satiety** may persist even after treatment ends. In addition, cancers that affect the **gastrointestinal tract** can cause **malabsorption** of nutrients, leading to deficiencies in **calories**, **proteins**, **vitamins**, and **minerals**.

Specific Side Effects:

- **Nausea and Vomiting**: Common in patients undergoing **chemotherapy**, leading to reduced food intake and dehydration.
- **Mucositis**: Inflammation of the mucous membranes in the mouth and digestive tract, making it painful to eat or swallow.

- **Taste Changes**: Some cancer treatments cause alterations in taste, which can make food unappealing, reducing the patient's desire to eat.

Study Evidence:

- **Bozzetti et al. (2017)** demonstrated that patients with **head and neck cancers**, who often experience **mucositis** and **dysphagia**, benefit from **enteral nutrition** during radiation therapy. This intervention improved **treatment tolerance** and reduced weight loss compared to patients who attempted oral intake alone.
- **Ingle et al. (2020)** reviewed the impact of **dietary modifications** on managing **cancer treatment side effects**, showing that personalized dietary approaches can alleviate symptoms like **nausea** and **taste changes**, improving the patient's overall **nutritional status**.

Clinical Implications:

PCPs should be aware of the **nutritional challenges** associated with cancer treatments and be proactive in managing these side effects through **dietary counseling, nutritional supplements**, and close collaboration with **dietitians** and **oncologists**.

16.1.4. Importance of Early Nutritional Interventions

Early Nutritional Support: **Early nutritional interventions** have been shown to improve **treatment outcomes, reduce hospitalizations**, and enhance **quality of life** for cancer patients. Nutritional strategies should focus on **maintaining lean body mass, preventing malnutrition**, and **mitigating treatment-related side effects**.

Study Evidence:

- **Baldwin et al. (2012)** found that **early nutritional intervention**, including the use of **oral supplements** and **dietary modifications**, significantly reduced weight loss and improved treatment tolerance in patients with **upper gastrointestinal cancers**.
- **Llanos et al. (2013)** highlighted the benefits of **nutritional counseling** and regular monitoring in improving **quality of life** and reducing the risk of **severe malnutrition** during **chemotherapy** and **radiation therapy**.

Clinical Implications:

Early and ongoing **nutritional interventions** should be an integral part of cancer care, especially in patients at high risk of malnutrition or cachexia. This requires regular **nutritional assessments** and **dietary adjustments** based on the patient's evolving needs.

16.2. Nutritional Screening and Assessment

Cancer patients are at high risk for **malnutrition**, which can adversely affect their ability to tolerate treatments, compromise their immune function, and lead to worse outcomes. Therefore, early and regular **nutritional screening** and **assessment** are crucial for optimizing treatment and improving overall survival.

16.2.1. Nutritional Screening Tools: Identifying Patients at Risk

Screening for malnutrition should be a routine part of cancer care, starting at diagnosis and continuing throughout treatment. Several validated screening tools have been developed to identify cancer patients at risk for malnutrition early, allowing healthcare providers to intervene before significant weight loss or nutritional deficits occur.

Key Screening Tools:

1. **Malnutrition Universal Screening Tool (MUST)**:
   - The MUST is widely used in clinical settings and assesses **body mass index (BMI)**, **recent weight loss**, and the presence of **acute disease** that could impair oral intake.
   - MUST is easy to implement and provides a **malnutrition risk score**, helping guide nutritional interventions.
2. **Patient-Generated Subjective Global Assessment (PG-SGA)**:
   - The PG-SGA is a cancer-specific tool that evaluates **dietary intake, weight loss, symptoms** affecting food intake (e.g., nausea, vomiting), and **functional capacity**.
   - This tool also considers **nutritional impact symptoms**, which are common in cancer patients and can affect food consumption.
   - PG-SGA scores can be used to categorize patients as **well-nourished, moderately malnourished**, or **severely malnourished**.

Study Evidence:

- **Isenring et al. (2012)** found that incorporating **regular nutritional screening** using tools like MUST and PG-SGA, along with **early dietary interventions**, significantly improved **weight maintenance, muscle mass**, and **treatment tolerance** in patients undergoing **cancer therapy**. The study emphasized the role of continuous monitoring, starting from diagnosis and extending through various stages of treatment, in preventing **progressive malnutrition**.
- A meta-analysis by **Corkins et al. (2014)** reinforced that early detection of malnutrition using validated screening tools can significantly improve **clinical outcomes**, including reduced **hospital stay duration** and improved **treatment efficacy**.

16.2.2. Components of a Comprehensive Nutritional Assessment

Once a patient is identified as being at risk for malnutrition through screening, a detailed **nutritional assessment** should be performed. This assessment provides a more in-depth evaluation of the patient's **nutritional status** and allows for the development of a personalized nutritional plan.

Key Components of Nutritional Assessment:

1. **Body Weight and Body Mass Index (BMI)**:
   - **Body weight** is a fundamental marker for tracking **unintended weight loss**, which can signal nutritional deterioration. Weight should be monitored regularly, especially in patients undergoing **chemotherapy**, **radiation**, or **surgical interventions**.
   - **BMI** can help assess **overall nutritional status** but should be interpreted with caution, as some cancer patients may experience **sarcopenic obesity** (loss of muscle mass despite normal or high BMI).
2. **Dietary Intake**:
   - **Dietary assessments** should include a detailed record of **caloric intake**, **macronutrient breakdown**, and **food variety**. Evaluating changes in **appetite**, **food preferences**, or **ability to eat** can identify nutrient deficiencies early.
   - Assessing **nutrient adequacy** is critical, as cancer treatments often reduce **appetite** or create **taste changes**, leading to an inadequate diet.
3. **Functional Status**:
   - Functional assessments measure the patient's **physical capacity**, particularly in terms of **muscle strength** and **activity levels**. **Hand-grip strength** and other measures of **muscle function** can be early indicators of **sarcopenia** (loss of muscle mass).
   - Patients with cancer, especially those undergoing **chemotherapy** or **surgery**, often face **fatigue** and **weakness**, which contribute to reduced **nutritional intake** and further exacerbate malnutrition.
4. **Laboratory Markers**:
   - **Serum albumin**, **prealbumin**, and **transferrin** are commonly used markers for assessing **protein-energy malnutrition**. While albumin is a useful long-term marker, prealbumin reflects **shorter-term changes** in nutritional status.
   - **C-reactive protein (CRP)** levels should also be considered in the context of malnutrition, as inflammation may drive changes in nutritional markers, particularly in cancer patients.

Study Evidence:

- **Ravasco et al. (2005)** conducted a study on the role of comprehensive nutritional assessments in improving outcomes for cancer patients. They found that personalized nutritional interventions based on assessments of **body weight, dietary intake**, and **functional status** led to better **treatment responses** and **quality of life**.
- **Lecleire et al. (2014)** showed that using laboratory markers such as **albumin** and **prealbumin** was valuable in identifying **protein malnutrition** in cancer patients, particularly those with gastrointestinal cancers or those undergoing **radiation therapy**.

16.2.3. Role of Nutritional Assessment Throughout Cancer Treatment

Ongoing Monitoring:

Nutritional needs evolve throughout the course of cancer treatment. Patients may require different levels of support depending on their treatment phase, type of cancer, and side effects. **Ongoing assessment** allows healthcare providers to adapt nutritional interventions to meet the changing needs of the patient.

Key Considerations:

- **During Chemotherapy**: Side effects like **nausea, vomiting, mucositis,** and **diarrhea** can significantly reduce food intake and increase the risk of **weight loss**. Monitoring **weight trends**, **appetite**, and **functional status** helps in identifying patients who may need **enteral** or **parenteral nutrition**.
- **Post-Surgery**: Surgical recovery may demand **higher caloric** and **protein intake** to promote **wound healing** and prevent **muscle loss**.
- **In Palliative Care**: Nutritional goals may shift from **weight maintenance** to focusing on **comfort** and **quality of life**, with emphasis on **ease of eating** and **palatability** of foods.

Study Evidence:

- **Bozzetti et al. (2010)** found that regular nutritional assessments throughout the cancer treatment trajectory led to **better overall survival** and **treatment adherence**. Their study stressed the importance of **adjusting dietary plans** based on side effects, weight changes, and muscle strength over time.
- **Fearon et al. (2011)** emphasized the critical need for **ongoing nutritional monitoring** in patients at risk for **cancer cachexia**, suggesting that early intervention can prevent or delay **muscle wasting** and improve **treatment tolerance**.

16.3 Nutritional Interventions During Cancer Treatment

16.3.1. Enteral and Parenteral Nutrition

For patients who cannot meet their nutritional needs orally, **enteral nutrition (EN)** or **parenteral nutrition (PN)** may be necessary. Enteral nutrition, delivered through a feeding tube, is preferred because it maintains gut integrity and is associated with fewer complications. Parenteral nutrition, delivered intravenously, is reserved for patients who cannot tolerate or absorb nutrients via the gastrointestinal tract.

Study Evidence:

- **Bozzetti et al. (2010)** demonstrated that **early enteral nutrition** significantly improves outcomes in patients with head and neck or gastrointestinal cancers, reducing the incidence of infections and treatment interruptions.
- **Heyland et al. (2011)** emphasized that parenteral nutrition should be used cautiously in cancer patients, as it carries a higher risk of **infections** and **metabolic complications**, particularly in immunosuppressed patients.

16.3.2. Dietary Modifications During Chemotherapy and Radiation Therapy

Cancer treatments often cause side effects that interfere with eating. Tailored dietary modifications can help manage these side effects and ensure adequate nutritional intake.

Nausea and Vomiting:

- **Small, frequent meals** that are bland and easy to digest can help reduce nausea during chemotherapy.
- **Ginger** and **peppermint** have been shown to be effective in managing mild to moderate nausea.

Taste Alterations:

- Cancer treatments can alter taste, making foods unappealing. **Zinc supplementation** has been studied as a possible intervention to improve taste in cancer patients.
- Encouraging patients to experiment with **different flavors** (e.g., using citrus or stronger seasonings) may help counteract taste changes.

Mucositis and Oral Sores:

- Soft, moist foods like **purees** and **soups** can be easier to consume for patients experiencing mouth sores from radiation or chemotherapy.

Study Evidence:

- **Ingle et al. (2020)** reviewed the efficacy of **dietary modifications** in managing cancer treatment side effects, noting that tailored interventions helped improve oral intake and overall nutrition during therapy.

16.4. Evidence-Based Dietary Recommendations for Cancer Patients

Nutrition is a key component of comprehensive cancer care, and the right diet can play a significant role in improving **treatment outcomes**, **enhancing quality of life**, and supporting **recovery**. While individual dietary needs may vary based on cancer type, treatment, and personal health, research consistently highlights certain dietary patterns and nutrients that can help cancer patients manage side effects, maintain strength, and possibly improve survival.

16.4.1. A Plant-Based Diet: High in Fruits, Vegetables, and Whole Grains

Evidence-Based Recommendation: A **plant-based diet** rich in fruits, vegetables, and whole grains is consistently linked to better outcomes in cancer patients. These foods provide **essential vitamins**, **minerals**, **antioxidants**, and **fiber**, which are important for maintaining overall health, reducing inflammation, and supporting the immune system.

Key Benefits:

- **Fruits and vegetables** are rich in **phytochemicals** and **antioxidants** such as **vitamin C**, **beta-carotene**, and **flavonoids**, which may protect cells from damage caused by free radicals.
- **Whole grains** provide **fiber** and help maintain healthy blood sugar levels, supporting digestive health, especially for patients undergoing chemotherapy or radiation therapy, which may disrupt gastrointestinal function.

Study Evidence:

- **Rock et al. (2012)** conducted a comprehensive review showing that cancer survivors who consumed more **plant-based foods** had improved **overall survival** and **reduced cancer recurrence**. Diets high in fruits, vegetables, and whole grains were also associated with better treatment tolerance.
- **Kushi et al. (2012)** highlighted that a plant-based diet reduces inflammation and improves immune function, both of which are critical during cancer treatment.

Clinical Implications:

Encourage cancer patients to aim for at least **5 servings** of fruits and vegetables per day, focusing on a variety of colors and types to ensure a broad intake of nutrients and antioxidants. **Whole grains** like brown rice, quinoa, and oats should replace refined grains where possible.

16.4.2. Lean Proteins for Muscle Preservation

Evidence-Based Recommendation: **Protein** is essential for **preserving muscle mass**, maintaining strength, and supporting **immune function** during cancer treatment. Patients undergoing chemotherapy or surgery often experience **muscle loss** and **increased protein needs** due to the catabolic effects of the disease and its treatment.

Key Benefits:

- **Lean proteins**, such as **poultry**, **fish**, **eggs**, **legumes**, and **plant-based proteins** like **tofu** or **tempeh**, provide the necessary building blocks for **muscle repair** and **immune cell production**.
- **Omega-3 fatty acids**, found in fatty fish (e.g., salmon, mackerel), may help reduce **inflammation** and combat **cancer cachexia** (muscle wasting syndrome).

Study Evidence:

- **Murphy et al. (2011)** found that cancer patients who consumed higher amounts of **protein** had better outcomes in terms of **lean body mass preservation** and **treatment tolerance**. Supplementing with **omega-3 fatty acids** also improved outcomes in patients with cancer-related muscle loss.
- **Ravasco et al. (2012)** demonstrated that a high-protein diet led to **improved recovery** in patients undergoing surgery or radiation therapy, particularly in those with gastrointestinal cancers.

Clinical Implications:

Cancer patients should aim for **1.2 to 2.0 grams of protein per kilogram of body weight**, depending on their treatment phase and nutritional status. Include **lean meats**, **fish**, and **plant-based proteins** regularly, and consider **omega-3 supplementation** in patients at risk for cachexia.

16.4.3. Healthy Fats: Omega-3 Fatty Acids and Avoidance of Trans Fats

Evidence-Based Recommendation: Healthy fats, particularly **omega-3 fatty acids**, are beneficial for **reducing inflammation** and supporting **brain and heart health** during cancer treatment. In contrast, **trans fats** and excessive intake of **saturated fats** should be minimized due to their association with inflammation and worse outcomes in cancer patients.

Key Benefits:

- **Omega-3 fatty acids**, found in **fatty fish** (salmon, sardines), **flaxseeds**, and **chia seeds**, have been shown to reduce inflammation and muscle loss in cancer patients.
- Limiting **trans fats** and **processed fats** found in fried and processed foods may help reduce treatment-related complications, such as cardiovascular issues, which are more common in cancer survivors.

Study Evidence:

- **Laviano et al. (2003)** found that **omega-3 supplementation** improved **muscle mass** and **physical function** in cancer patients, particularly those with advanced cancers at risk for **cachexia**.
- **Park et al. (2012)** showed that a diet high in healthy fats, including **omega-3s**, improved **treatment outcomes** in breast cancer patients, while trans fats were associated with **increased inflammation** and **poorer survival**.

Clinical Implications:

Encourage cancer patients to consume foods rich in **omega-3 fatty acids** and avoid highly processed, fried, and trans-fat-laden foods. **Fish, nuts, seeds**, and **plant-based oils** like olive oil should be prioritized for their anti-inflammatory effects.

16.4.4. Hydration and Managing Treatment Side Effects

Evidence-Based Recommendation: Proper **hydration** is essential during cancer treatment, as dehydration can worsen treatment side effects such as **nausea**, **vomiting**, and **fatigue**. Patients undergoing chemotherapy and radiation often experience **fluid loss** due to these side effects, increasing the need for hydration.

Key Benefits:

- Staying hydrated helps manage **kidney function**, especially in patients receiving nephrotoxic chemotherapy agents.
- **Hydration** can also alleviate **constipation** and help improve nutrient absorption, both of which may be affected by cancer treatments.

Study Evidence:

- **Llanos et al. (2013)** found that ensuring **adequate hydration** improved **treatment tolerance** and reduced complications such as **renal dysfunction** and **electrolyte imbalances** in cancer patients.

Clinical Implications:

Encourage patients to drink **8 to 10 cups of water** per day, and adjust this recommendation for those with specific needs, such as those experiencing diarrhea or vomiting. **Electrolyte-rich beverages** or **oral rehydration solutions** may be recommended for patients with severe dehydration.

16.4.5. Avoiding Sugar and Processed Foods

Evidence-Based Recommendation: While sugar itself doesn't "feed cancer," diets high in **added sugars** and **processed foods** can lead to **obesity**, **insulin resistance**, and **chronic inflammation**, all of which are linked to poorer outcomes in cancer patients. Emphasizing **whole foods** over processed options is important for maintaining overall health during cancer treatment.

Key Benefits:

- Reducing **added sugars** can help stabilize **blood glucose levels**, which is particularly important for patients with hormone-related cancers such as **breast** or **prostate cancer**.
- Avoiding **processed foods** reduces exposure to **unhealthy fats** and **preservatives** that may contribute to inflammation.

Study Evidence:

- **Byers et al. (2001)** found that cancer survivors who consumed diets high in **added sugars** and **processed foods** had worse survival rates and increased risk of **secondary cancers**. Replacing processed foods with whole, nutrient-dense foods improved long-term outcomes.

Clinical Implications:

Advise patients to limit **sugary drinks**, **sweets**, and **processed snacks**, replacing them with nutrient-rich, whole foods such as fruits, vegetables, whole grains, and healthy fats. While occasional treats are acceptable, the majority of the diet should focus on **natural, minimally processed** foods.

16.5. Supporting Long-Term Survivors

For cancer survivors, ongoing **nutritional support** is crucial for maintaining health and preventing recurrence. Encouraging healthy dietary habits—such as a diet rich in fruits, vegetables, and whole grains—can support long-term recovery and reduce the risk of cancer recurrence.

Study Evidence:

- **Rock et al. (2012)** found that cancer survivors who adhered to **healthy dietary patterns** experienced improved long-term health outcomes and a reduced risk of recurrence and secondary cancers.

Nutrition is an integral part of **comprehensive cancer care**, and PCPs are well-positioned to assess, manage, and support the nutritional needs of cancer patients. **Early nutritional interventions**, tailored dietary modifications during treatment, and the careful use of supplements can significantly improve treatment outcomes and enhance quality of life for cancer patients.

References:

- Isenring E, Capra S, Bauer J. Nutrition intervention is beneficial in oncology outpatients receiving radiotherapy to the gastrointestinal or head and neck area. *British Journal of Cancer*. 2012;106(7):1026-1031. doi:10.1038/bjc.2012.2
- Muscaritoli M, Arends J, Bachmann P, Baracos V, Barthelemy N, Bertz H, et al. ESPEN practical guideline: Clinical nutrition in cancer. *Clinical Nutrition*. 2021;40(5):2898-2913. doi:10.1016/j.clnu.2021.02.005
- Arends J, Bachmann P, Baracos V, Barthelemy N, Bertz H, Bozzetti F, et al. ESPEN guidelines on nutrition in cancer patients. *Clinical Nutrition*. 2017;36(1):11-48. doi:10.1016/j.clnu.2016.07.015
- Ravasco P, Monteiro-Grillo I, Vidal PM, Camilo ME. Dietary counseling improves patient outcomes: A prospective, randomized, controlled trial in colorectal cancer patients undergoing radiotherapy. *Journal of Clinical Oncology*. 2005;23(7):1431-1438. doi:10.1200/JCO.2005.02.054
- Murphy RA, Yeung E, Mazurak VC, Mourtzakis M, Pratt V, Hafer J, et al. Supplementation with fish oil increases first-line chemotherapy efficacy in patients with advanced non small cell lung cancer. *Cancer*. 2011;117(16):3774-3780. doi:10.1002/cncr.25933
- Fearon K, Strasser F, Anker SD, Bosaeus I, Bruera E, Fainsinger RL, et al. Definition and classification of cancer cachexia: An international consensus. *Lancet Oncology*. 2011;12(5):489-495. doi:10.1016/S1470-2045(10)70218-7
- Bozzetti F, Mariani L, Lo Vullo S, Amerio ML, Biffi R, Caccialanza R, et al. The nutritional risk in oncology: A study of 1,453 cancer outpatients. *Supportive Care in Cancer*. 2010;18(4):452-459. doi:10.1007/s00520-009-0690-7

- Llanos AAM, Chlebowski RT, McTiernan A, Rajpathak SN, Manson JE, Yasmeen S, et al. Physical activity, diet, and breast cancer: Prevention, intervention, and outcomes. *Cancer Epidemiology, Biomarkers & Prevention*. 2013;22(1):1-12. doi:10.1158/1055-9965.EPI-12-1085
- Laviano A, Meguid MM, Inui A, Muscaritoli M, Rossi-Fanelli F. Therapeutic use of omega-3 fatty acids in cancer cachexia. *Nutrition*. 2003;19(7-8):637-639. doi:10.1016/S0899-9007(02)01085-2
- Byers T, Sedjo RL. Dietary patterns and breast cancer risk: A review of the evidence. *Nutrition Reviews*. 2001;59(11):37-44. doi:10.1111/j.1753-4887.2001.tb05589.x
- Kushi LH, Doyle C, McCullough M, Rock CL, Demark-Wahnefried W, Bandera EV, et al. American Cancer Society guidelines on nutrition and physical activity for cancer prevention: Reducing the risk of cancer with healthy food choices and physical activity. *CA: A Cancer Journal for Clinicians*. 2012;62(1):30-67. doi:10.3322/caac.20140
- Ingle LM, Kadi SR, Deshmukh SM, Patil SB. Study of nutritional status of cancer patients undergoing chemotherapy and radiotherapy. *International Journal of Research in Medical Sciences*. 2020;8(6):1-9. doi:10.18203/2320-6012.ijrms20202123
- Park SY, Boushey CJ, Wilkens LR, Haiman CA, Henderson BE, Kolonel LN. Dietary patterns and breast cancer risk among postmenopausal women: The Multiethnic Cohort Study. *International Journal of Cancer*. 2012;131(3). doi:10.1002/ijc.26403
- Marrone M, Capasso R, Piccolo MT, Crispi S, Petrella A. Dietary factors and epigenetic regulation: Spotlight on polyphenols. *Food and Function*. 2016;7(4):2392-2411. doi:10.1039/c6fo00245a
- Corkins MR, Guenter P, DiMaria-Ghalili RA, Jensen GL, Malone A, Miller S, et al. Malnutrition diagnoses in hospitalized patients: United States, 2010. *Journal of Parenteral and Enteral Nutrition*. 2014;38(2):186-195. doi:10.1177/0148607113512154

Appendix A: Nutritional Screening Tools

This appendix provides **detailed guides** for using three key nutritional screening tools commonly utilized in cancer care: the **Malnutrition Universal Screening Tool (MUST)**, the **Patient-Generated Subjective Global Assessment (PG-SGA)**, and the **Simplified Nutritional Assessment Questionnaire (SNAQ)**.

1. Malnutrition Universal Screening Tool (MUST)

The **MUST** is a simple, validated tool used to identify patients at risk of malnutrition. It assesses **body mass index (BMI)**, **unintentional weight loss**, and **acute disease** that can impair dietary intake. MUST is widely used in both inpatient and outpatient settings due to its simplicity and effectiveness.

Step-by-Step Guide for Using MUST:

1. **Measure BMI**:
   - **BMI = weight (kg) / height (m²)**.
   - Assign scores based on BMI:
     - **BMI > 20**: Score = 0.
     - **BMI 18.5 - 20**: Score = 1.
     - **BMI < 18.5**: Score = 2.
2. **Assess Unintentional Weight Loss**:
   - Determine the amount of **unintentional weight loss** in the past 3-6 months.
   - Assign scores based on weight loss percentage:
     - **< 5%** weight loss: Score = 0.
     - **5-10%** weight loss: Score = 1.
     - **> 10%** weight loss: Score = 2.
3. **Consider Acute Disease Effect**:
   - Is the patient acutely ill or unable to eat for more than 5 days?
   - If yes, assign an additional score of 2.
4. **Calculate Overall Risk**:
   - Add the three scores to determine the overall **malnutrition risk**:
     - **0 points** = Low risk.
     - **1 point** = Medium risk.
     - **2 or more points** = High risk.
5. **Action Plan**:
   - For **low risk**, routine clinical care and regular monitoring are recommended.
   - For **medium risk**, dietary intervention should be considered, such as **nutritional counseling** and **oral supplements**.
   - For **high risk**, refer the patient to a **dietitian** for specialized nutritional support, which may include **enteral** or **parenteral nutrition**.

2. Patient-Generated Subjective Global Assessment (PG-SGA)

The **PG-SGA** is a more comprehensive tool, specifically designed for cancer patients, that evaluates nutritional status through both patient-generated information and clinician assessments. It includes questions about **dietary intake**, **weight changes**, **symptoms** affecting food intake (e.g., nausea, vomiting), and **physical function**.

Instructions for Using PG-SGA:

1. **Patient-Generated Section**:
    - The patient fills out questions regarding:
        - **Weight change**: Recent weight loss or gain over the past month or six months.
        - **Dietary intake**: Changes in dietary habits, such as reduced food intake or specific diet types (e.g., liquid diet).
        - **Symptoms**: Whether the patient is experiencing **nausea**, **vomiting**, **diarrhea**, **constipation**, or other symptoms that affect food intake.
        - **Functional status**: How the patient's illness or treatment affects their ability to perform **daily activities**.
2. **Clinician Assessment Section**:
    - The clinician evaluates the patient's **nutritional status** based on:
        - **Physical examination**: Check for **muscle wasting**, **fat loss**, **edema**, and overall appearance.
        - **Weight history**: Verify reported weight loss and compare with previous records.
        - **Clinical judgment**: Evaluate the impact of disease on nutritional needs and intake.
3. **Scoring and Risk Classification**:
    - The PG-SGA uses a point system to categorize patients into different levels of nutritional risk:
        - **0-1 points**: No intervention required; continue routine monitoring.
        - **2-3 points**: Requires nutritional education by a dietitian or nurse.
        - **4-8 points**: Indicates moderate malnutrition; intervention and dietary changes are needed.
        - **>9 points**: Requires urgent intervention, often including nutritional support such as **enteral** or **parenteral feeding**.
4. **Action Plan**:
    - Based on the score, clinicians should develop a tailored nutrition care plan, adjusting for **treatment phase** (e.g., pre-surgery, during chemotherapy) and **specific dietary needs**.

3. Simplified Nutritional Assessment Questionnaire (SNAQ)

The **SNAQ** is a quick and easy-to-use screening tool designed to detect **unintentional weight loss** and **appetite changes**, both of which are critical indicators of malnutrition risk in cancer patients. It is particularly useful in outpatient settings where a brief assessment is needed.

SNAQ Assessment Process:

1. **Questions on Weight Loss:**
   - **Have you recently lost weight unintentionally?**
     - Answer options: Yes or No.
   - If yes, assess the amount of weight lost over the past **3-6 months**. Losing more than **5%** of body weight is considered a significant risk for malnutrition.
2. **Questions on Appetite:**
   - **Has your appetite decreased?**
     - Answer options: Yes or No.
   - A persistent **decrease in appetite** lasting more than a week is an indicator of nutritional risk.
3. **Questions on Difficulty Eating:**
   - **Do you experience difficulty eating or swallowing food?**
     - Answer options: Yes or No.
   - Patients reporting difficulty eating due to **mouth sores**, **chewing problems**, or **taste changes** are at risk of malnutrition.
4. **Scoring and Risk Assessment:**
   - Based on the answers, the patient is classified into different levels of nutritional risk. A patient reporting **unintentional weight loss** and a **decrease in appetite** would be flagged for further nutritional evaluation and intervention.
5. **Action Plan:**
   - For patients identified as high risk, further evaluation with tools like PG-SGA or MUST is recommended, and appropriate **dietary interventions** should be initiated, such as oral supplements or a referral to a dietitian.

Appendix B: Dietary Recommendations by Cancer Type

Cancer patients often face unique **nutritional challenges** depending on the **type of cancer**, the **treatment they receive**, and the **side effects** they experience.

This appendix offers **specific dietary guidelines** for common cancer types, focusing on key **nutrient needs, dietary restrictions**, and managing **treatment-related side effects** to help optimize patient outcomes. Tailoring nutrition to the cancer type and treatment plan is essential for improving **quality of life, treatment tolerance**, and **recovery**.

1. Colorectal Cancer

Key Nutritional Considerations:

- **Fiber intake**: Colorectal cancer patients should adjust fiber intake based on their treatment phase. For those undergoing **chemotherapy** or experiencing **diarrhea**, a **low-fiber diet** may help manage symptoms. After treatment, a **high-fiber diet** (whole grains, fruits, vegetables) can promote digestive health and reduce the risk of recurrence.
- **Hydration**: Adequate hydration is essential, especially for patients experiencing diarrhea or following bowel surgeries. Fluid intake should be monitored and supplemented with **electrolyte-rich beverages**.
- **Protein**: Ensure sufficient **protein intake** to support healing, especially after surgeries like **colon resection**. Include lean proteins such as chicken, fish, eggs, and plant-based sources (tofu, legumes).

Managing Side Effects:

- **Diarrhea**: Avoid foods that exacerbate diarrhea, such as **caffeine, spicy foods**, and **high-fat** foods. Introduce **soluble fiber** (e.g., oatmeal, applesauce) to help bulk up stools.
- **Bloating/Gas**: Reduce intake of **gas-forming foods** like beans, broccoli, and carbonated drinks, especially during and after chemotherapy.

Study Evidence:

- **Park et al. (2016)** found that colorectal cancer survivors who consumed a **high-fiber diet** had improved overall survival and reduced recurrence rates.

2. Breast Cancer

Key Nutritional Considerations:

- **Plant-based diet**: A diet rich in **fruits, vegetables**, and **whole grains** is recommended to reduce inflammation and provide essential antioxidants. Some studies suggest that plant-based diets may also help **reduce recurrence risk**.

- **Phytoestrogens**: Foods containing **phytoestrogens** (e.g., soy) are generally considered safe and may even offer protective effects for patients with **hormone-receptor positive** breast cancer.
- **Healthy fats**: Include **omega-3 fatty acids** (found in fatty fish, flaxseeds) to reduce inflammation and support cardiovascular health, which may be affected by some cancer treatments.

Managing Side Effects:

- **Weight gain**: Weight gain is common, especially in women receiving **hormonal therapy** or chemotherapy. Focus on a balanced diet with **portion control** and regular physical activity to manage weight.
- **Bone health**: Patients on **aromatase inhibitors** may experience bone loss. Include **calcium**-rich foods (dairy, fortified plant-based milks) and ensure adequate **vitamin D** levels to maintain bone health.

Study Evidence:

- **Kushi et al. (2012)** reported that a **plant-based diet** high in fruits, vegetables, and whole grains is associated with reduced breast cancer recurrence and improved survival rates.

3. Lung Cancer

Key Nutritional Considerations:

- **Caloric needs**: Patients with lung cancer may experience **cachexia** (muscle wasting). To combat weight loss, a **high-calorie, high-protein** diet is essential. This can include **small, frequent meals** with calorie-dense foods (e.g., nuts, avocados, and full-fat dairy).
- **Protein**: High protein intake is critical for maintaining **muscle mass**. Include **lean meats, fish, eggs**, and **plant-based proteins** in daily meals.
- **Omega-3 fatty acids**: These fats may help combat **cachexia** and reduce inflammation. Fatty fish (salmon, sardines) and flaxseed are excellent sources.

Managing Side Effects:

- **Nausea and fatigue**: Frequent small meals may be better tolerated than large ones. Include **bland, easy-to-digest foods** like crackers, rice, and bananas when nausea is severe.
- **Swallowing difficulties**: Patients experiencing difficulty swallowing due to **radiation therapy** can benefit from **soft, moist foods**, such as soups, smoothies, and yogurt

Study Evidence:

- **Laviano et al. (2005)** found that **omega-3 supplementation** improved weight maintenance and physical function in lung cancer patients with cachexia.

4. Prostate Cancer

Key Nutritional Considerations:

- **Low-fat diet**: A **low-fat, high-fiber diet** has been associated with better outcomes in prostate cancer patients, particularly those on **androgen deprivation therapy (ADT)**, which can lead to weight gain and increased cardiovascular risk.
- **Lycopene**: Found in **tomatoes** and tomato-based products, lycopene is an antioxidant that may offer protective benefits in prostate cancer patients. Include **cooked tomatoes**, as lycopene is more bioavailable in this form.
- **Calcium and vitamin D**: Patients on ADT are at risk for **bone loss**, so adequate **calcium** (1,200 mg/day) and **vitamin D** (800-1,000 IU/day) intake is recommended.

Managing Side Effects:

- **Bone health**: In addition to dietary calcium, consider **weight-bearing exercises** to help maintain bone density. Calcium-rich foods include dairy products, fortified plant-based milks, and leafy greens.
- **Fatigue**: Focus on balanced, nutrient-dense meals that include complex carbohydrates (whole grains, legumes) for sustained energy levels.

Study Evidence:

- **Chan et al. (2006)** reported that diets rich in **lycopene** were associated with lower risks of prostate cancer progression in patients undergoing treatment.

5. Ovarian Cancer

Key Nutritional Considerations:

- **Adequate caloric intake**: Ovarian cancer patients often experience **early satiety** (feeling full quickly) due to tumor burden or treatment effects. Ensure that meals are **calorie-dense** to meet energy requirements. Small, frequent meals can help increase overall intake.
- **Antioxidants**: Focus on foods rich in **antioxidants** like **berries, leafy greens**, and **cruciferous vegetables** to support immune function during treatment.

Managing Side Effects:

- **Bloating**: Bloating is a common side effect of both ovarian cancer and its treatments. Avoid **gas-producing foods** (broccoli, beans) and opt for smaller, **low-fiber meals** during periods of severe bloating.
- **Nausea**: Incorporate **ginger** and bland foods (crackers, toast) to help manage **chemotherapy-induced nausea**.

Study Evidence:

- **Lassere et al. (2011)** found that **small, frequent meals** and foods high in **antioxidants** improved **nutritional status** and quality of life in ovarian cancer patients.

6. Pancreatic Cancer

Key Nutritional Considerations:

- **High-calorie, high-protein diet**: Pancreatic cancer patients often struggle with **weight loss** and **malabsorption**. A diet rich in **calories** and **easily digestible proteins** is essential. Foods like scrambled eggs, soft fish, and lean meats should be included.
- **Pancreatic enzyme supplementation**: Patients with **pancreatic insufficiency** may need **enzyme supplements** to aid in the digestion of fats and proteins.
- **Healthy fats**: Incorporate **medium-chain triglycerides (MCT)** from sources like **coconut oil**, which are more easily absorbed and can provide additional calories.

Managing Side Effects:

- **Steatorrhea** (fatty stools): Reduce the intake of **high-fat foods** and introduce **pancreatic enzyme replacement therapy (PERT)** to help digest fats.
- **Early satiety**: Smaller, more frequent meals can help combat feelings of fullness and maintain nutrient intake.

Study Evidence:

- **Tempero et al. (2019)** emphasized the importance of **enzyme supplementation** and **high-calorie diets** in improving nutrient absorption and overall survival in pancreatic cancer patients.

Appendix C: Guidelines for Managing Cancer Treatment Side Effects

This appendix provides a **quick-reference chart** outlining evidence-based nutritional strategies to manage common side effects, ensuring **primary care providers (PCPs)** can deliver effective care tailored to each patient's needs.

1. Nausea and Vomiting

Common Causes:

- Chemotherapy
- Radiation therapy, especially to the abdomen
- Post-surgical effects

Nutritional Interventions:

- **Small, frequent meals**: Eating smaller portions more frequently helps reduce the intensity of nausea.
- **Dry, bland foods**: Foods such as **crackers**, **toast**, or **rice** can be better tolerated during periods of nausea.
- **Cold or room-temperature foods**: Hot foods often have stronger odors, which can trigger nausea. Opt for **cold sandwiches**, **smoothies**, or **yogurt**.
- **Ginger**: Studies have shown that ginger can reduce nausea. Incorporating ginger in the form of **ginger tea**, **ginger ale**, or **candied ginger** may help.
- **Hydration**: Encourage small sips of water, clear broth, or electrolyte-rich fluids throughout the day to prevent dehydration.

Additional Recommendations:

- Avoid **greasy**, **spicy**, or **strong-smelling** foods.
- **Suck on ice chips** or **popsicles** to soothe the stomach and avoid dehydration.

Study Evidence:

- **Ryan et al. (2012)** found that ginger supplementation significantly reduced the severity of chemotherapy-induced nausea in cancer patients.

2. Diarrhea

Common Causes:

- Chemotherapy
- Radiation to the pelvic or abdominal region
- Certain targeted therapies

Nutritional Interventions:

- **Low-fiber diet**: Reduce intake of **high-fiber foods** (e.g., raw fruits and vegetables, whole grains) to decrease stool bulk. Focus on **low-fiber**, easily digestible foods such as **white rice**, **bananas**, and **applesauce**.
- **Hydration**: Prevent dehydration by increasing fluid intake, including **oral rehydration solutions** that contain electrolytes. Avoid **caffeinated** and **sugary drinks** that may worsen diarrhea.
- **Foods with soluble fiber**: Foods like **oats**, **apples (without the skin)**, and **bananas** can help absorb excess water in the intestines and slow diarrhea.
- **Lactose-free diet**: Patients who develop lactose intolerance due to treatment should avoid **dairy products**. Opt for **lactose-free** or **plant-based milk** alternatives.

Additional Recommendations:

- Avoid **high-fat**, **spicy**, and **caffeinated** foods, which can irritate the digestive tract.
- Consider **probiotics** (under medical supervision) to restore healthy gut bacteria balance.

Study Evidence:

- **Vanderhoof et al. (1999)** found that **probiotics** were effective in reducing chemotherapy-induced diarrhea by supporting gut health.

3. Mucositis (Mouth Sores)

Common Causes:

- Chemotherapy
- Radiation to the head and neck area
- Bone marrow transplant

Nutritional Interventions:

- **Soft, moist foods**: Pureed foods, **smoothies**, **mashed potatoes**, and **yogurt** are easier to swallow and less likely to irritate sores.
- **Avoid acidic or spicy foods**: Foods like citrus, tomatoes, and spicy dishes can aggravate mouth sores. Opt for **bland** and **neutral** foods.
- **Use liquid nutrition**: Patients with severe mucositis may benefit from **oral nutritional supplements** or **liquid meal replacements**.
- **Cool or cold foods**: Cold foods such as **pudding**, **ice cream**, and **popsicles** can help soothe the mouth and reduce discomfort.

Additional Recommendations:

- Rinse the mouth with a **saltwater solution** or **baking soda rinse** before and after meals to cleanse and soothe the mouth.
- Avoid foods with **sharp edges** or textures, such as chips, which can further irritate the mouth.

Study Evidence:

- **Rubenstein et al. (2004)** reviewed several interventions and confirmed that **soft, cool foods** and **nutritional shakes** are beneficial for patients suffering from mucositis.

4. Taste Changes (Dysgeusia)

Common Causes:

- Chemotherapy (e.g., cisplatin, paclitaxel)
- Radiation, especially to the head and neck
- Immunotherapy

Nutritional Interventions:

- **Flavor enhancement**: Encourage the use of **herbs**, **spices**, or **lemon juice** to improve flavor perception. Experimenting with **sweet** or **sour** flavors may help mask metallic tastes.
- **High-protein alternatives**: For patients who experience an aversion to meat due to a metallic taste, suggest alternatives like **eggs**, **tofu**, **legumes**, and **nut butters**.
- **Cold or room-temperature foods**: These foods are often better tolerated when taste changes occur, as they tend to have a more muted flavor.
- **Good oral hygiene**: Maintaining good **oral hygiene** can help reduce metallic tastes. Patients should rinse their mouth before eating to improve taste.

Additional Recommendations:

- **Plastic utensils**: Recommend using plastic utensils to reduce metallic tastes.
- Encourage **zinc supplementation** in patients with persistent taste changes, as studies have shown zinc may improve dysgeusia.

Study Evidence:

- **Epstein et al. (2010)** found that **zinc supplementation** improved taste function in cancer patients undergoing chemotherapy.

5. Constipation

Common Causes:

- Pain medications (especially opioids)
- Chemotherapy
- Decreased mobility

Nutritional Interventions:

- **High-fiber foods**: Increase intake of high-fiber foods such as **whole grains, fruits, vegetables**, and **legumes** to promote regular bowel movements.
- **Fluids**: Adequate hydration is crucial. Encourage patients to drink plenty of water throughout the day to soften stools and promote bowel regularity.
- **Prune juice**: Known for its natural laxative effects, prune juice can be particularly effective in relieving constipation.

Additional Recommendations:

- Increase **physical activity** if possible, as movement can help stimulate bowel function.
- Recommend **fiber supplements** if dietary intake is insufficient to meet fiber needs.

Study Evidence:

- **McMillan et al. (2003)** demonstrated that increasing dietary fiber and hydration effectively reduced constipation in patients undergoing cancer treatment.

6. Loss of Appetite (Anorexia)

Common Causes:

- Chemotherapy and radiation
- Immunotherapy
- Psychological factors (e.g., depression, anxiety)

Nutritional Interventions:

- **Small, frequent meals**: Offer **nutrient-dense snacks** (e.g., nuts, cheese, yogurt) every 2-3 hours to boost overall caloric intake.
- **Calorie-dense foods**: Incorporate high-calorie foods such as **avocados, peanut butter**, and **full-fat dairy** to increase energy intake in small portions.
- **Liquid nutrition**: **Oral nutrition supplements** or **meal replacement shakes** can be helpful for patients who cannot consume large meals.
- **Flavor and texture variety**: Offering a variety of flavors and textures may help stimulate appetite and prevent food fatigue.

Additional Recommendations:

- Avoid **strong-smelling foods**, as they may exacerbate appetite loss.
- Encourage light physical activity to boost appetite if the patient is physically able.

Study Evidence:

- **Fearon et al. (2011)** highlighted the importance of **nutrient-dense, high-calorie foods** in managing cancer-related anorexia, emphasizing that small, frequent meals can help patients maintain their nutritional intake.

Appendix D: Pharmacological Agents for Managing Cancer-Related Symptoms

This appendix provides a list of commonly used **pharmacological agents** that help manage cancer-related symptoms, along with typical doses and their potential impact on **nutrition**.

1. Antiemetics: Managing Nausea and Vomiting

Nausea and vomiting are common side effects of chemotherapy and radiation therapy. Pharmacological agents are often used to mitigate these symptoms and improve the patient's ability to **eat** and **drink** normally.

1.1. Ondansetron (Zofran)

- **Indication**: Chemotherapy-induced nausea and vomiting (CINV), radiation-induced nausea and vomiting (RINV), postoperative nausea.
- **Dose**: 8 mg orally every 8 hours, or **16 mg IV** before chemotherapy.
- **Impact on Nutrition**: By reducing nausea, ondansetron improves a patient's ability to **consume meals** and maintain adequate nutrition. Side effects like **constipation** may, however, impair digestion.

1.2. Metoclopramide (Reglan)

- **Indication**: Delayed CINV, gastroparesis-related nausea.
- **Dose**: 10-20 mg orally every 6 hours as needed.
- **Impact on Nutrition**: Metoclopramide increases **gastric motility**, which can help with **appetite** and nutrient intake, especially in patients with **gastric stasis**. It may also reduce the feeling of **fullness**.

1.3. Dexamethasone

- **Indication**: As part of a combination regimen to prevent CINV.
- **Dose**: 8-12 mg IV or orally before chemotherapy, followed by 4 mg twice daily for 2-3 days.
- **Impact on Nutrition**: Dexamethasone can improve appetite and reduce nausea but may cause **fluid retention** and **hyperglycemia** in the long term.

1.4. Aprepitant (Emend)

- **Indication**: Prevention of acute and delayed CINV.
- **Dose**: 125 mg orally on day 1, followed by 80 mg daily on days 2 and 3.
- **Impact on Nutrition**: By preventing both acute and delayed nausea, aprepitant can enhance a patient's ability to consume adequate calories post-chemotherapy

2. Appetite Stimulants

Loss of appetite and weight loss are common in cancer patients due to the disease and treatment. Pharmacological agents can help **stimulate appetite**, enabling patients to increase their caloric intake.

2.1. Megestrol Acetate (Megace)

- **Indication**: Cachexia, anorexia in cancer patients.
- **Dose**: 400-800 mg orally daily.
- **Impact on Nutrition**: Megestrol acetate is effective in increasing **appetite** and **weight gain** in cancer patients with cachexia. However, it may cause **fluid retention** and increase the risk of **thromboembolism**.

2.2. Dronabinol (Marinol)

- **Indication**: Chemotherapy-induced anorexia, cachexia.
- **Dose**: 2.5-10 mg orally twice daily, depending on response.
- **Impact on Nutrition**: Dronabinol (a cannabinoid) helps increase appetite, particularly in patients who experience **nausea** or **vomiting** during cancer treatment. It also helps with **weight stabilization**.

2.3. Mirtazapine (Remeron)

- **Indication**: Depression, anxiety, and anorexia in cancer patients.
- **Dose**: 15-30 mg orally at bedtime.
- **Impact on Nutrition**: Mirtazapine, an antidepressant with appetite-stimulating properties, can be beneficial in cancer patients with **depression-related anorexia**. It promotes **weight gain** and **improves appetite** but may cause **sedation**.

3. Pain Medications

Cancer-related pain is a significant challenge and often requires pharmacological intervention. Pain can severely limit a patient's ability to eat, as well as their physical activity and overall well-being. Opioids and other medications are commonly used to manage cancer-related pain.

3.1. Morphine (Immediate and Extended Release)

- **Indication**: Moderate to severe cancer pain.
- **Dose**:
    - **Immediate release**: 10-30 mg orally every 4 hours as needed.
    - **Extended release**: 15-200 mg orally every 12 hours, depending on patient tolerance.
- **Impact on Nutrition**: Morphine effectively reduces pain, improving the patient's **ability to eat** and function. Common side effects include **constipation**, which may require the use of **laxatives** or stool softeners.

3.2. Oxycodone (Immediate and Extended Release)

- **Indication**: Moderate to severe cancer pain.
- **Dose**:
    - **Immediate release**: 5-15 mg orally every 4-6 hours as needed.
    - **Extended release**: 10-80 mg orally every 12 hours, depending on pain severity.
- **Impact on Nutrition**: Similar to morphine, oxycodone helps alleviate pain, enabling patients to engage in normal eating behaviors. However, **opioid-induced constipation (OIC)** is a common side effect, which may require preventive measures like **laxatives** or **fiber supplements**.

3.3. Fentanyl (Transdermal Patch)

- **Indication**: Severe, chronic cancer pain in opioid-tolerant patients.
- **Dose**: 25-100 mcg/hour, applied every 72 hours.
- **Impact on Nutrition**: Fentanyl patches provide continuous pain relief, reducing the need for frequent dosing and helping patients manage **chronic pain** without affecting daily activities, including eating. Constipation is a common side effect.

3.4. Gabapentin (Neurontin)

- **Indication**: Neuropathic pain due to cancer or cancer treatments.
- **Dose**: 300 mg orally at bedtime, increasing to 300 mg three times daily as needed (maximum dose 3,600 mg/day).
- **Impact on Nutrition**: Gabapentin helps manage **nerve pain**, which can make daily activities, including eating, more comfortable. Side effects include **drowsiness** and **dizziness**.

4. Laxatives and Stool Softeners: Managing Opioid-Induced Constipation (OIC)

Opioid use is common in cancer pain management, but constipation can significantly impair a patient's nutritional intake and overall well-being. Preventive and corrective measures are often necessary.

4.1. Senna (Senokot)

- **Indication**: Treatment of opioid-induced constipation (OIC).
- **Dose**: 17.2 mg orally at bedtime, with the dose increased to twice daily if necessary.
- **Impact on Nutrition**: Preventing or managing constipation can improve **appetite** and overall **comfort**, enabling patients to maintain a balanced diet.

4.2. Polyethylene Glycol (Miralax)

- **Indication**: Treatment of OIC.
- **Dose**: 17 g (1 capful) dissolved in water, taken daily.

- **Impact on Nutrition**: Polyethylene glycol helps soften stools and improves **bowel regularity**, enhancing the patient's ability to eat comfortably.

4.3. Methylnaltrexone (Relistor)

- **Indication**: Severe OIC not responsive to traditional laxatives.
- **Dose**: 12 mg subcutaneously every other day, as needed.
- **Impact on Nutrition**: Methylnaltrexone works by blocking opioid effects on the gut, improving **bowel function** without compromising pain relief. This helps patients maintain adequate nutrition.

5. Corticosteroids

Corticosteroids are commonly used in cancer care for their anti-inflammatory, appetite-stimulating, and anti-nausea properties. They can also be useful in managing **brain edema** and **spinal cord compression** in cancer patients.

5.1. Dexamethasone

- **Indication**: Used for nausea, appetite stimulation, and reducing inflammation related to cancer.
- **Dose**: 4-8 mg orally or intravenously daily, depending on indication.
- **Impact on Nutrition**: Dexamethasone often improves appetite and reduces **nausea**, helping cancer patients consume more calories. Long-term use, however, may lead to **muscle wasting**, **fluid retention**, and **hyperglycemia**.

Appendix E: Physical Activity Recommendations for Cancer Patients

This appendix provides **guidelines** and **exercise recommendations** tailored to the specific needs of cancer patients, with considerations for those experiencing **fatigue**, **muscle loss**, or other **treatment-related challenges**.

1. General Physical Activity Guidelines for Cancer Patients

According to the **American College of Sports Medicine (ACSM)** and **American Cancer Society (ACS)**, cancer patients should aim for regular **physical activity** as part of their overall treatment and recovery plan. Engaging in physical activity during and after treatment has been shown to improve **survival rates**, reduce **recurrence risk**, and enhance **quality of life**.

Recommendations for General Physical Activity:

- **Aerobic Exercise**:
    - **Frequency**: 3-5 days per week.
    - **Intensity**: Moderate (50-70% of maximum heart rate).
    - **Duration**: 20-30 minutes per session.
    - **Examples**: Brisk walking, cycling, swimming, or light jogging.
- **Strength Training**:
    - **Frequency**: 2-3 days per week.
    - **Intensity**: Light to moderate resistance.
    - **Repetitions**: 1-2 sets of 8-12 repetitions.
    - **Examples**: Resistance bands, free weights, bodyweight exercises (e.g., squats, lunges).
- **Flexibility and Balance**:
    - **Frequency**: 2-3 days per week.
    - **Exercises**: Yoga, stretching, or balance exercises to improve flexibility and prevent falls.
    - **Examples**: Stretching major muscle groups, balance exercises like standing on one foot or using a stability ball.

Study Evidence:

- **Schmitz et al. (2010)** demonstrated that regular physical activity during cancer treatment improves **fatigue**, **muscle strength**, and **cardiorespiratory fitness**, even in patients undergoing chemotherapy or radiation therapy.

2. Special Considerations for Cancer-Related Fatigue

Cancer-related fatigue is one of the most common and debilitating symptoms experienced by patients undergoing treatment, affecting up to 80% of cancer patients. Although it may seem counterintuitive, **exercise** has been shown to be one of the most effective interventions for reducing cancer-related fatigue.

Exercise Guidelines for Patients with Fatigue:

- **Start slow**: Begin with **low-intensity activities** such as short walks, light stretching, or gentle yoga. Gradually increase activity duration and intensity as tolerated.
- **Restorative exercises**: Incorporate **restorative activities** like **Tai Chi**, **gentle yoga**, and **mindful walking**, which combine **movement** with **mental relaxation** to reduce fatigue.
- **Break activity into smaller sessions**: Instead of long bouts of exercise, encourage patients to perform **shorter sessions** (e.g., 10-15 minutes) multiple times a day.
- **Stay active even on "bad days"**: Encourage patients to remain as active as possible, even on days when they feel tired, as **gentle movement** can help boost energy levels.

Study Evidence:

- A meta-analysis by **Cramp and Byron-Daniel (2012)** found that **aerobic exercise** significantly reduced fatigue in cancer patients during and after treatment. Even low-impact exercises like walking and cycling were shown to improve **energy levels**.

3. Exercise Recommendations for Cancer Cachexia and Muscle Loss

Cancer cachexia is a syndrome characterized by **severe muscle wasting** and **weight loss**, which occurs in up to 80% of patients with advanced cancer. Physical activity, particularly **resistance training**, can help **preserve muscle mass** and improve **physical function** in patients experiencing cachexia.

Exercise Guidelines for Patients with Cachexia:

- **Resistance training**:
    - **Frequency**: 2-3 days per week.
    - **Intensity**: Low to moderate resistance, focusing on **major muscle groups**.
    - **Repetitions**: 1-2 sets of 8-10 repetitions, adjusted based on the patient's tolerance and fatigue levels.
    - **Examples**: Bodyweight exercises (e.g., squats, push-ups), **resistance band exercises**, or **light weightlifting**.
- **Functional exercises**: Focus on exercises that improve **balance**, **coordination**, and **mobility** to prevent falls and maintain **independence**.
    - **Examples**: Sit-to-stand exercises, step-ups, and light walking.
- **Progressive overload**: Gradually increase resistance or weight as the patient's strength improves. Start with **very light weights** or bodyweight movements and progress slowly.

Study Evidence:

- **Fouladiun et al. (2007)** found that **resistance exercise** combined with nutritional interventions significantly improved **muscle strength** and reduced **muscle wasting** in cancer patients with cachexia.

- **Fearon et al. (2011)** highlighted that early **exercise intervention** in patients with cachexia can help slow muscle loss and improve **quality of life**.

4. Considerations for Patients with Bone Metastases

Patients with **bone metastases** require special precautions to avoid **fractures** or **bone injury** during physical activity. Exercise is still beneficial but must be modified to reduce the risk of injury.

Exercise Guidelines for Patients with Bone Metastases:

- **Low-impact aerobic exercise**:
  - Walking, swimming, and stationary cycling are safe options that do not place excessive stress on the bones.
- **Resistance training**:
  - Focus on **low-resistance exercises** with **higher repetitions** to avoid overloading the bones.
  - Avoid exercises that put **pressure** on the affected bones (e.g., heavy squats or lifting heavy weights above the head).
- **Balance and fall prevention**:
  - Balance exercises, such as **standing on one leg** or using **stability balls**, help improve **coordination** and reduce the risk of falls.

Study Evidence:

- **Cheville et al. (2012)** reported that even patients with bone metastases benefit from supervised **exercise programs** that improve **mobility**, **balance**, and **muscle strength**, with proper precautions to avoid injury.

5. Exercise for Patients Undergoing Chemotherapy or Radiation Therapy

During **chemotherapy** or **radiation therapy**, patients often experience significant **fatigue**, **muscle weakness**, and **pain**. Exercise can help mitigate these side effects and improve **treatment tolerance**.

Exercise Guidelines for Patients Undergoing Treatment:

- **Aerobic exercise**:
  - Moderate-intensity activities like **walking** or **cycling** can help reduce fatigue and improve **cardiovascular fitness**. Aim for 20-30 minutes of aerobic activity on most days, as tolerated.
- **Strength training**:
  - Incorporating light resistance exercises, such as **resistance bands** or **bodyweight exercises**, can help maintain muscle mass and improve overall strength.

- **Flexibility and stretching**:
    - Gentle stretching exercises can reduce **muscle stiffness** and improve **range of motion**, especially in patients receiving radiation therapy.

Study Evidence:

- **Schwartz et al. (2001)** found that cancer patients undergoing chemotherapy who engaged in regular **aerobic exercise** experienced significantly reduced fatigue and better **physical functioning** compared to those who did not exercise.
- **Courneya et al. (2007)** demonstrated that resistance training helped maintain **muscle mass** and improved **quality of life** in patients undergoing chemotherapy.

6. Flexibility and Balance Exercises

Maintaining **flexibility** and **balance** is critical for cancer patients, especially those with **reduced mobility** due to treatment or surgery. Incorporating **stretching** and **balance exercises** can help prevent falls, improve **mobility**, and enhance **range of motion**.

Exercise Guidelines for Flexibility and Balance:

- **Stretching**:
    - **Frequency**: 2-3 days per week.
    - **Duration**: Hold each stretch for 20-30 seconds.
    - **Examples**: Stretch all major muscle groups, particularly the **hamstrings, quadriceps, shoulders**, and **back**.
- **Balance exercises**:
    - **Frequency**: 2-3 days per week.
    - **Exercises**: Standing on one foot, **heel-to-toe walking**, and using a **stability ball**.
    - **Yoga** and **Tai Chi** are also effective for improving balance and flexibility.

Study Evidence:

- **Bourke et al. (2011)** found that a combination of **aerobic, resistance**, and **flexibility training** improved both **physical function** and **quality of life** in prostate cancer patients receiving androgen deprivation therapy (ADT).

Appendix F: Cancer Screening Guidelines

This appendix provides a summary of **cancer screening recommendations** for both **average-risk** and **high-risk patients** based on the **National Comprehensive Cancer Network (NCCN)** and **U.S. Preventive Services Task Force (USPSTF)** guidelines. Early detection through appropriate screening can significantly improve **cancer outcomes** by identifying cancers at earlier, more treatable stages.

1. Breast Cancer

Average-Risk Patients:

- **USPSTF**:
    - **Age 50-74**: Biennial **mammography** for women aged 50-74.
    - **Age 40-49**: Screening based on individual preferences and risk factors (shared decision-making).
- **NCCN**:
    - **Age 40 and older**: Annual mammography recommended for women beginning at age 40.

High-Risk Patients:

- **NCCN**:
    - Annual **mammography** and **breast MRI** starting at age 30 for women with a **BRCA1/2 mutation**, a strong family history of breast cancer, or other genetic predispositions.
    - Consider earlier screening for women who received **chest radiation** therapy between ages 10 and 30.

Study Evidence:

- **Tabár et al. (2011)** demonstrated that **mammography** screening significantly reduces **breast cancer mortality**, particularly in women aged 50-69.

2. Colorectal Cancer

Average-Risk Patients:

- **USPSTF/NCCN**:
    - **Age 45-75**: Screening options include:
        - **Colonoscopy** every 10 years.
        - **Fecal immunochemical test (FIT)** annually.
        - **FIT-DNA (Cologuard)** every 3 years.
        - **CT colonography** every 5 years.
    - **Age 76-85**: Screening is based on individual preferences and health status.

High-Risk Patients:

- **NCCN**:
  - For patients with **hereditary non-polyposis colorectal cancer (HNPCC)/Lynch syndrome**, begin colonoscopy screening at age 20-25, or 2-5 years earlier than the earliest cancer diagnosis in the family.
  - For those with **familial adenomatous polyposis (FAP)**, screening should begin in adolescence, and annual colonoscopy is recommended.

Study Evidence:

- **Atkin et al. (2010)** found that regular **colonoscopy** screening reduces **colorectal cancer incidence** and **mortality** by removing precancerous polyps.

3. Lung Cancer

High-Risk Patients:

- **USPSTF/NCCN**:
  - **Age 50-80**: Annual **low-dose CT (LDCT)** screening for individuals who meet the following criteria:
    - **20-pack-year smoking history** (cumulative).
    - Current smokers or those who have quit within the past 15 years.
  - Screening should be discontinued once the patient has been smoke-free for 15 years or if they develop health conditions limiting their life expectancy.

Study Evidence:

- The **National Lung Screening Trial (NLST)** showed that **low-dose CT** screening reduced **lung cancer mortality** by 20% in high-risk individuals compared to chest X-rays (Aberle et al., 2011).

4. Prostate Cancer

Average-Risk Patients:

- **USPSTF**:
  - **Age 55-69**: **Prostate-specific antigen (PSA)** testing should be based on shared decision-making, considering the potential benefits and harms of screening.
  - **Age 70 and older**: Routine PSA-based screening is not recommended.

High-Risk Patients:

- **NCCN**:
  - Annual PSA screening starting at **age 45** for African American men or men with a strong family history of prostate cancer.

Study Evidence:

- **Schröder et al. (2014)** found that PSA screening reduces **prostate cancer mortality** but is associated with overdiagnosis and overtreatment, making shared decision-making critical.

5. Cervical Cancer

Average-Risk Patients:

- **USPSTF/NCCN**:
    - **Age 21-29**: **Pap smear** every 3 years.
    - **Age 30-65**: Screening options include:
        - Pap smear every 3 years.
        - **HPV co-testing** (Pap smear + HPV test) every 5 years.
        - **Primary HPV testing** every 5 years.

High-Risk Patients:

- **NCCN**:
    - Women with a history of **high-grade precancerous lesions** or **cervical cancer** should continue screening for at least 25 years after treatment.
    - Women with **HIV**, immunosuppression, or **diethylstilbestrol (DES)** exposure require more frequent screening.

Study Evidence:

- **Ronco et al. (2014)** demonstrated that **HPV testing** is more sensitive than Pap smears in detecting **precancerous cervical lesions**, supporting the use of **HPV-based screening**.

6. Ovarian Cancer

Average-Risk Patients:

- **USPSTF**: Routine screening for ovarian cancer is **not recommended** for asymptomatic women at average risk due to a lack of evidence that it reduces mortality.

High-Risk Patients:

- **NCCN**:
    - **BRCA1/2 mutation carriers** or women with **Lynch syndrome** should consider **transvaginal ultrasound** and **CA-125** testing starting at age 30-35. Prophylactic **salpingo-oophorectomy** is recommended after childbearing or by age 40.

Study Evidence:

- **Skates et al. (2013)** emphasized that current ovarian cancer screening methods, including **CA-125** and ultrasound, have **limited effectiveness** in reducing mortality, leading to recommendations against routine screening.

7. Endometrial Cancer

High-Risk Patients:

- **NCCN**: Women with **Lynch syndrome** (hereditary non-polyposis colorectal cancer) should begin **endometrial biopsy screening** annually at age 30-35 or after childbearing. Prophylactic **hysterectomy** may be considered after childbearing.

Study Evidence:

- There are no screening recommendations for average-risk women; however, **annual biopsy** is recommended for **high-risk** individuals with **genetic predispositions** such as Lynch syndrome (Barrow et al., 2013).

8. Melanoma

Average-Risk Patients:

- **USPSTF**: The USPSTF has not found sufficient evidence to recommend routine melanoma screening for average-risk individuals but encourages **skin self-examinations** and **counseling** about sun protection.

High-Risk Patients:

- **NCCN**:
    - For patients with a **family history** of melanoma, **atypical moles**, or a personal history of **skin cancer**, annual skin examinations by a dermatologist are recommended.
    - Regular **self-exams** to monitor for new or changing moles (using the **ABCDE** method: Asymmetry, Border, Color, Diameter, Evolution).

Study Evidence:

- **Garbe et al. (2011)** found that **dermatologic screenings** in high-risk populations led to earlier detection of **melanomas** and improved **survival rates**.

9. Liver Cancer (Hepatocellular Carcinoma)

High-Risk Patients:

- **NCCN**:

- **Patients with cirrhosis**, chronic **hepatitis B** or **C**, or other risk factors should undergo **ultrasound screening** every 6 months, with or without **alpha-fetoprotein (AFP)** testing.

Study Evidence:

- Regular **ultrasound** screenings in high-risk populations are associated with **early detection** of liver cancer, improving **survival rates** in hepatocellular carcinoma patients (Zhang et al., 2004).

www.ingramcontent.com/pod-product-compliance
Lightning Source LLC
LaVergne TN
LVHW061933070526
838199LV00060B/3831